# HOW TO LOVE

# MIDLIFE

## Unlocking **15** Reasons To Loving Life In Your Golden Years

Amber N. Spruill

# Table of content

**Falling In Love With Midlife**

**Falling In Love With Midlife**

# Introduction

Have you ever wondered if you still have the best extended periods of your life ahead of you? Imagine living a life in which every moment is treasured, every day brings something fresh to the table, and the wisdom of your experience illuminates the path ahead. Greetings from midlife, a time often misunderstood but full of promise and fulfillment.

Moments of pure bliss sprinkled across life, often arising out of nowhere and leaving just as swiftly. If these happy moments are not appreciated, they run the risk of being overlooked amidst the daily flurry of activity. Our days are full of countless blessings that we usually take for granted, from the sun's rays to the laughter we share with those we love. Recognizing and appreciating these small but important moments, sharing a laugh, thinking back on a fond memory, seeing our children succeed, or finishing a difficult task is essential to falling in love with midlife.

According to brain science, midlife can be a stressful and existentially uncertain time. However, it can also be a period of unparalleled clarity and assurance. Many in their 50s and 60s say they feel happier and more content with life than they have in the past. Falling in Love with Midlife inspires you to approach this phase of your life with gratitude and purpose.

Permit me to tell you a short tale. Imagine a 47-year-old woman named Clara who decided to revisit her childhood dream of becoming a painter. Clara had spent many years raising a family, working in a corporate setting, and hardly ever taking time for herself.

One beautiful evening, while organizing her storage area, she just so happened to come across an old, dusty easel and a paint case. She placed them on her lawn as opposed to throwing them away. which started as a reluctant brushstroke and quickly developed into a creative explosion. Lost in a world of variations and memories, Clara ended up painting for quite some time. Her family noticed another sparkle in her eyes, and she had a deep sense of fulfillment that had been lacking for a very long time. Clara's narrative exemplifies the joy that comes from rekindling old passions and welcoming fresh experiences in middle age.

Midlife is a time to take stock of your life and adjust it to better suit your true self. It's a chance to say no to things that no longer serve you and yes to aspirations that have been in your heart. This deliberate way of living promotes contentment and happiness. Ongoing education and self-awareness prevent the stagnation sometimes associated with midlife crises, turning this phase into a journey of self-discovery.

**Falling In Love With Midlife**

A vital component of falling in love with midlife is one's health. A lively, happy existence is enhanced by eating healthily, remaining active, and fostering prosperity. It's never too late to adopt healthy habits, as demonstrated by stories of sluggish people who take great pleasure in shocking real achievements.

Consider the example of Clara's 94-year-old uncle, who decided to compete in a long-distance race at the age of 90. Along with finishing the race, he received a decoration specific to his age group. When he told the family about his victory, his face lit up with unmatched joy, demonstrating that age is nothing more than a number when it comes to living out your dreams.

It becomes essential as we become older to think about how we should gracefully and intelligently transition into the next phase of our lives. How to Love in Midlife challenges you to appreciate the here and now, concentrate on your success, and discover joy in the simple, pleasant moments of everyday life. Thus, pick up that paintbrush, scuff up those running shoes, and fall madly in love with the joy that life offers! This is your guide to making midlife a journey filled with excitement and possibility.

This book will reveal the top 15 reasons to embrace life during your golden years and provide advice on how to elevate the ordinary to the extraordinary. Open a copy of Falling in Love with Midlife to learn how to turn these years into the most rewarding time of your life. Every justification serves as a springboard for realizing the brilliance and promise of midlife. You will discover practical advice and motivation to further your path, whether it's rekindling previous passions, creating new connections, or discovering novel experiences.

# PHYSICAL LIFE

# Chapter One

## How Can I Prioritize Physical Health and Wellness?

Midlife essentialness, energy, and overall personal pleasure depend on concentrating on true well-being and health. Our bodies undergo many changes as we age, and adopting a proactive approach to wellness might make it easier for us to explore these changes. These are the important steps and phases to concentrate on real health and happiness in midlife.

***Adopt the Standard Real labor***: For what purpose does it matter? Regular exercise is essential for mental health, physical health, flexibility, and strength of muscles. It can help reduce the risk of chronic illnesses such as diabetes, osteoporosis, and heart disease.

- Choose an Activity You Enjoy: Choose activities that you find appealing, such as walking, swimming, cycling, yoga, or dancing. This increases the likelihood that you will remain with them.

- Consolidate Strength Training: To maintain bone thickness and bulk, incorporate opposing workouts at least twice a week. Weightlifting, resistance training, and body-weight exercises like squats and push-ups might all fall under this category.

- Continue to be Trustworthy: Aim for 150 minutes per week of moderate-to-high power oxygen-consuming exercise or 75 minutes per week of high-intensity exercise combined with muscle-reinforcing exercises.

***Pay Attention to Complete Wellbeing***: For what purpose does it matter? A balanced diet provides the necessary nutrients to support bodily functions, maintain energy levels, and prevent diet-related illnesses.

- Consume a Variety of Foods: Include a range of organic goods, veggies, whole grains, lean meats, and healthy fats in your diet. This ensures that you receive a variety of supplements.

- Control Parts: To avoid overindulging, be mindful of portion sizes. It can be helpful to use smaller plates and to be aware of your body's signals of cravings.

- Stay Hydrated: Throughout the day, sip a lot of water. Sufficient hydration maintains cognitive function, energy levels, and overall health.

***Get Enough Sleep***: For what purpose does it matter? Good sleep is essential for mental clarity, physical well-being, and strong bonds with family members. It allows the body to heal and regenerate.

- Establish a daily routine: Even on the weekends, go to bed and wake up at the same time every day. This regulates the internal clock of your body.

- Create a Climate: Make sure your room is a cool, quiet, and relaxing place to sleep. Invest in comfortable couches and beds.

- Cap Energizers: Avoid heavy meals, caffeine, and nicotine right before bed. If everything else is equal, engage in relaxing pursuits like reading or contemplation.

***Routine Health Examinations and Preventive Measures***: For what purpose does it matter? Regular examinations and screenings help identify possible health issues early on when they are easier to treat.

- Schedule Standard Check-Ups: For routine physical examinations, circulatory strain assessments, cholesterol checks, and other age-appropriate testing, see your medical services provider.

- Remain Up to Date on Immunizations: Make sure you receive any recommended vaccinations, such as the shingles vaccine, influenza shot, and others, as advised by your healthcare physician. Screen Constant Circumstances: Adhere to your treatment plan and have regular screenings for any pre-existing conditions, such as diabetes or hypertension.

***See Pressure Firsthand***: For what purpose does it matter? Persistent pressure can harm overall health, exacerbating illnesses such as heart disease, depression, and impaired susceptibility.

- Put Relaxation Techniques into Practice: Engage in activities that promote relaxation, such as deep breathing exercises, yoga, or introspection.
- Stay Connected: Maintain your strong points in your relationships with your family, friends, and neighborhood. Strong

relationships can relieve stress and provide significant assistance.

- Pursue side interests: Put effort into pursuits you find fulfilling. Engaging in hobbies can be a fantastic way to decompress and rejuvenate.

***Avoid Adopting Painful Habits***: For what purpose does it matter? Reducing or eliminating harmful behaviors can significantly improve your quality of life and longevity.

- Quit Smoking: If you smoke, seek assistance in quitting. The medical benefits of quitting smoking are both immediate and long-term.

- Limiting Alcohol: Enjoy alcohol restraint. This means that women are reliant on one drink per day, whereas males can have up to two drinks per day.

## What kinds of activities can help me stay fit and active?

Midlife wellness, mental health, and overall personal pleasure are all dependent on maintaining an active and healthy lifestyle. Including a variety of exercises in your routine will help you maintain a good level of strength, flexibility, adaptability, and cardiovascular health. These are some specific suggestions and benefits of engaging in healthy, active hobbies.

### *Energy-dense exercise*

For what purpose does it matter? Cardio, or oxygen-consuming exercise, improves cardiovascular health, lung capacity, endurance, and weight management. It releases endorphins, which can improve mood and alleviate stress.

- Trolling: This is a simple, low-impact activity that ought to be feasible everywhere. Spend at least thirty minutes per day, five days a week, going after the gold. When strolling is done with friends or family, it can be a social activity.

- Running: Running can fundamentally assist cardiovascular well-being for those who engage in more intense activity. Start small and gradually increase your miles.

- Cycling: Cycling is a fantastic way to improve cardiovascular health and leg strength, whether you do it outside or on an exercise bike. Moreover, it is easier on the joints than running.

- Swimming: Provides a full-body workout with negligible impact on joints. Perseverance, muscular strength, and cardiovascular health can all be enhanced by swimming.

- movement: In addition to being social and amusing, movement helps improve cardiovascular health, balance, and coordination. Think about taking a dance class or simply dancing at home to your favorite song.

### *Exercise for Strength*

For what purpose does it matter? Strength training maintains mass, improves overall physical strength, supports digestion, and works on bone thickness. It's especially important because mass typically decreases with age.

- Powerlifting: Make use of obstacle groups, weight machines, or freeloads. Concentrate on large muscle groups such as the arms, back, legs, and chest. Aim for the highest three weekly strength training sessions.

- Weightlifting Exercises: Anywhere should be able to perform push-ups, squats, rushes, and boards without the need forequipment. These workouts can improve flexibility, balance, and strength even more.

- Groups in Opposition: Blockage groups are small and adaptable and can be used for a broad range of exercises targeting different muscle groups.

- Pilates: A low-impact training system that emphasizes body shaping, flexibility, and center strength. Similarly, Pilates helps enhance posture and balance.

### Training for Equilibrium and Adaptability

For what purpose does it matter? Exercises focusing on balance and adaptability can prevent injuries, enhance posture, and increase daily functioning. They are essential for maintaining adaptability and lowering the risk of falls.

- Yoga: Combines physical postures, breathing techniques, and introspection. Yoga improves flexibility, balance, strength, and clarity of mind. Yoga comes in a variety of forms, from the gentle Hatha to the more dynamic Vinyasa or Power Yoga.

- Judo: A military art form characterized by deliberate, deliberate movements and deep relaxation. Judo is especially beneficial for more experienced adults since it enhances balance, flexibility, and mental focus.

- Extending: Include extending exercises in your regular practice sessions. Concentrate on large muscle groups and hold each stretch for 20 to 30 seconds. It should be possible to extend independently or following physical activity.

### *Athletic and Outdoor Activities*

For what purpose does it matter? Engaging in sports and outdoor activities can add variety to your fitness routine, enhance the enjoyment of exercise, and provide psychological and local benefits by connecting you with the natural world.

- Climbing: While engaging in outdoor activities, climbing provides an exceptional cardiovascular workout. Climbing on altered ground strengthens muscles and improves balance even more.

- Cultivating: A delightful way to be active. Bending, lifting, and stretching are examples of cultivating, which can improve flexibility and strength.

- Playing Sports: Sports like b-ball, tennis, or golf can provide a lighthearted and effective way to stay in shape. Enhancing social relationships can also be achieved by joining a local organization or club.

- Kayaking or paddleboarding: Excellent for building cardiovascular endurance and chest strength. Additionally, being in the water has a significant impact on the brain.

### Body-Mind Exercises

For what purpose does it matter? Mind-body exercises integrate physical development with relaxation techniques and mental focus. They help reduce stress, promote mental clarity, and enhance prosperity in general.

- Reflection: Regular practice of reflection can improve focus, lower stress levels, and enhance well-being at home. Combine with minimal real effort, such as strolling in contemplation.

- Qigong: A traditional Chinese form of meditation, breathing, and assisted development. Qigong can enhance one's abilities to maintain balance, adjust, and focus.

### Social and Get-Together Events

For what purpose does it matter? Participating in group practice can increase motivation, assign responsibilities, and improve enjoyment. Social cooperation during group activities also promotes mental and domestic well-being.

- Bunch Wellness programs: Enroll in Zumba, intense exercise, twist, or strength training programs at your local rec center or public space. These courses provide structured activities led by qualified instructors.

- Jogging or Strolling Groups: Participating in a group can inspire you and add charm to your workout. Moreover, it's a great opportunity to meet new people.

- Dance Classes: Learn about different dance genres such as salsa, assembly hall, and line dancing. These classes may be a fun way to stay active and social.

### Including Movement in Everyday Living

For what purpose does it matter? Small adjustments to your daily routine can raise your general action level without needing specific workout time.

- Make Use of the Stairwell: Whenever possible, take the stairs rather than the elevator. Walk or Bike for Short Outings: If possible, choose to walk or bike rather than drive to local objections.

- Stand and Move Frequently: Take advantage of breaks every hour to stand, stretch, and take a stroll if your job requires little physical exertion.

- Dynamic Family Tasks: Running errands for the family, such as vacuuming and cleaning, might count as real labor. To maximize the benefits of their involvement, make these assignments more engaging.

## In what way should I modify my diet to achieve optimal health?

Changing your diet for midlife optimal health is a comprehensive approach that considers your nutritional needs, way of life, and any existing medical conditions. Our bodies change with age, requiring different kinds of vitamins and having varied metabolic rates. These are specific steps to help you modify your diet for maximum health during your golden years.

### *Recognize Your Healthy Requirements*

For what purpose does it matter? Age-related changes in nutritional requirements are caused by factors such as bone thickness, mass, digestion, and the body's ability to absorb certain supplements. It is critical to comprehend these developments to maintain overall health.

- Speak with a Healthcare Professional: Determine your specific nutritional needs based on your lifestyle and health state by speaking with a specialist or a registered dietitian.
- Educate Yourself: Learn about the essential supplements that are important for midlife, such as fiber, protein, calcium, vitamin D, and healthy fats.

## *Pay Attention to All Food Types*

For what purpose does it matter? Whole food variants are little processed and rich in essential vitamins, fiber, and agents that prevent cancer, all of which contribute to overall wellness.

- Increased Ground-Grown Foods Admission: To ensure a range of nutrients and minerals, choose the best types available. Fresh, frozen, and canned foods (devoid of added salt or sugar) are excellent options.

- Choose Whole Grains: Rather than processed grains, choose whole grains like quinoa, whole wheat bread, oats, and earthy-colored rice. Whole grains are higher in vitamins and fiber.

- Add Nuts and Seeds: These are excellent sources of fiber, protein, and good fats. Serve them as a snack or add them to bowls of mixed greens or yogurts.

### *Keep Macronutrients Balanced*

For what purpose does it matter? A balanced intake of carbohydrates, proteins, and fats is essential for maintaining body weight, energy levels, and general health.

- Carbs: Choose complex carbohydrates such as whole grains, veggies, fruits that are organic, and vegetables. They are high in fiber and provide sustained energy.

- Proteins: Ensure that enough protein is admitted to maintain bulk. Include fish, eggs, dairy, vegetables, lean meats, and plant-based proteins like tempeh and tofu in your diet.

- Fats: Include heart-healthy fats from foods like almonds, avocados, olive oil, and fatty fish. Reduce saturated fats and avoid trans fats.

### *Put micronutrients front and center*

For what purpose does it matter? Minerals and other micronutrients are necessary for bodily functions like digestion, safe functioning, and bone health.

- Vitamin D and calcium are essential for healthy bones. Add dairy products, energizing plant-based milk, leafy vegetables, and fatty seafood. Whenever your primary care provider suggests an improvement, consider it.

- B Nutrients: Important for the production of energy and the health of the brain. Sources include whole grains, meats, poultry, dairy products, and salad greens.

- Reinforcements for cells: help combat oxidative stress and irritability. Consume a variety of vibrant plants, seeds, and nuts.

### Examine the piece sizes

For what purpose does it matter? Managing portion sizes helps maintain a healthy weight and prevent overindulgence when digestion slows down with age.

- Use More Modest Plates: This can help keep piece sizes under control without making you feel excluded.

- Recognize your appetite signals. Eat when you're hungry and quit when you're satisfied rather than full.

- Mindful Eating: During feasts, pay attention to what you eat, savor every bite, and avoid distractions like television or cell phones.

### *Drink plenty of water*

For what purpose does it matter? For processing, supplement absorption, and most bodily functions, enough hydration is essential. Dehydration can lead to a variety of health problems, including weakness and anxiety.

- Hydrate Frequently: Drink eight cups of water a day without holding back. This can include liquids, herbal teas, and foods high in water content, such as soil-derived goods.

- Limit Sweet Drinks: Steer clear of beverages with a lot of added sugar, such as soda and coffee-based drinks. If everything else is equal, choose water, herbal teas, or diluted natural product juices.

### Reduce Sodium Intake

For what purpose does it matter? Excessive intake of salt is linked to hypertension, which raises the risk of heart disease and stroke.

- Recognize Marks: Look up the sodium level of food names and choose options with less sodium.

- Cook at Home: Preparing meals at home gives you more control over the amount of salt you use.

- Use tastes and Spices: Instead of using salt to flavor your cuisine, try using citrus, spices, and tastes.

### Restrict added sugar intake

For what purpose does it matter? Consuming a lot of added sugars can lead to diabetes, weight gain, and heart disease.

- Avoid Sugary Snacks and Pastries: Choose healthy snacks like almonds, yogurt, or natural products.
- Pay close attention to the Fixings: Be aware of the added sugars in the sauces, toppings, and prepared food sources.
- Select Regular Sugars: Use regular sugars sparingly, such as honey or maple syrup.

### Nutritious Cooking Methods

For what purpose does it matter? The presence of harmful compounds and the health benefits of food can be affected by cooking methods.

- Opt for Healthier Methods: Instead of broiling, use steam, heat, barbecue, or sautéing. These techniques utilize less oil while preserving more nutrients.
- Limit Handled Food Sources: These often have high sodium content, added sugars, and harmful fats. When circumstances permit, settle on novel food varieties in their whole.

# Chapter Two

## Maintaining My Vitality and Energy

Everyone wants to age gracefully and maintain their physical health. Although it's common knowledge that age is just a number, there's rarely a moment at which neglecting your health is irreversible. Here are some fundamental tips to maintain your attractiveness and vitality as you get older.

### Maintaining an active body

Staying active as you age is essential to maintaining your wellness. Whatever the case, your peak years occur when your chemicals fizzle out and your body stops feeling like it. As we age, our testosterone levels decline, making it more difficult to maintain muscle mass and get in shape while belly fat grows.

**Falling In Love With Midlife**

Stay active by going to the rec center, working out at home, and running. However, focused energy workouts are not the total of well-being. Dance if, by some chance, you find it enjoyable to move! Maintaining your energy levels high, your joints healthy, and your pulse rate elevated are all related to practice. Consistency, not force, is the idea. Your body will recognize your worth for a considerable amount of time if you move it.

*Maintain your physical health*

You should take care of your body since it is your refuge. While it's not expected that you should give up your indulgences, maintaining a consistent eating schedule will help. Include in your diet bright, plant-based meals, entire grains, lean meats, and healthy fats.

Never forget that being hydrated is your best friend. Always have a water bottle with you. It's also important to remember that little, dark chocolate never does anyone any damage. Recall that you should concentrate on giving your body the vitamins it needs to grow rather than starving yourself.

*Accept responsibility*

Things can throw you curveballs in life, but how you handle them can determine a lot. Now is a great time to check in with stress as it may be a subtle guest. Accept self-care practices such as journaling, deep breathing, and introspection. Give up the things you cannot control and concentrate on the here and now. A healthy body results from a tranquil mind.Remember that the finest medicine for your soul is a good, hearty laugh!

*Establish strong ties*

Like the glue that binds us together, our buddies. Social partnerships are like a fantastic prescription drug for your well-being. Whether it's via phone conversations, coffee dates, or online home bases, stay in touch with your loved ones.Embrace the company of upbeat individuals who support and embrace your unique identity. Love, laughter, and shared experiences are the foundation of a substance heart.

### *Keep Yourself Hydrated*

Maintaining your energy levels and general health depends on drinking enough water. Never withhold more than 8 to 8 ounces of water each day, and increase your intake if you are exercising or exerting yourself in hot or dry conditions.Drink lots of drinks throughout the day to avoid being exhausted due to parchedness.

### *Concentrate on getting enough sleep*

The body ages and several cycles slow down, including the ability for self-healing. Your body can heal, regenerate, and reenergize itself as you sleep. Never deprive yourself of your nine hours of peaceful sleep each night. Establish a daily routine that includes a hot shower, some tea made at home, and some relaxing music. Turn off all of your electronics around an hour before bed, and create a relaxing sleeping environment to aid in falling asleep quickly. You'll wake up refreshed and prepared to tackle the day.

### Concentrate on looking after yourself

It's okay to put your needs first. Pay close attention as your body communicates what it needs. Take advantage of the three-day weekend if that's what you'd like. Make plans if you'd like to spend some alone time by the sea. Are there throbsin your joints? Find ways to correct it quickly before it deteriorates. Taking care of oneself is not selfish; rather, it is an essential component of living your greatest life.

### Uplift your complexion and overall look

The primary indicator of your vitality is the beauty of your skin. Therefore, remember it. As your skin becomes less dewy and smooth, moisturize it with rich creams. Your skin's natural radiance can be enhanced with a healthy diet and enough moisture.

### Schedule routine clinical examinations

**Falling In Love With Midlife**

Clinical examinations are crucial throughout life, but in your adult years, things can go wrong very quickly. Standard clinical tests allow you to identify potential problems before they become significant concerns. Make plans for annual physicals, exams, and screenings. Concentrating on these tests will ensure a healthy and uneventful journey through life.

*Midlife Nutritional Techniques to Boost Your Energy*

Given the abundance of conflicting information about what, when, and how to eat, it's easy to make a mistake and pursue comfort food. You need to be healthy and slim, regardless of whether you need to lose weight.

Your ability to digest food decreases with age. This suggests that you need less food because your energy requirements decrease. Sadly, it also suggests that your body is carrying extra weight, which you should be eager to shed. Whether we are dynamic or not, as we age, we often lose bulk, and our body's ability to absorb and utilize nutrients decreases.

Even while you can't stop these cycles from happening, you may lessen their effects by following and maintaining a supplement-rich diet and good nutrition practices. A few small adjustments will have a significant impact on bone health, the immune system, physical wellness, and much more.

## <u>Which nutritional approach is most effective for women over 50?</u>

Choosing the best method depends on your goals and way of living. You can see what your body requires when you know what you are trying to achieve. For example, if you are very new to exercise, your dietary needs will be different from those of someone training for a long-distance marathon!

Regardless of your current level, you can always start with the tactics below. These pointers can help you feel more positive and lead a better life!

## Consume more dense food sources and supplements.

Thick supplementation refers to regular, unprocessed, unrefined food types. It is advisable to include more of the following food varieties:

- Among the foods high in protein include eggs, egg whites, fish, poultry, turkey, lean hamburgers, buffalo, lentils, beans, and plain Greek yogurt.

- Foods high in sugars include beans and lentils, buckwheat, quinoa, sorghum, farro, millet, potatoes, kefir, plain Greek yogurt, new and frozen organic products, corn, and yams.

- Additional virgin olive oil, pecan oil, avocado oil, cheeses, nuts (cashews, pistachios, almonds, peanuts, and regular peanut butter), olives, pesto produced with olive oil, nut margarine from various classes, and seeds (chia, flax, hemp, pumpkin, and sesame)

- VEGETABLES: Indulge in a variety of colorful produce items such as tomatoes, radishes, eggplant, bell peppers, butternut squash, kale, cauliflower, broccoli, and red peppers, among others. In essence, consume the rainbow.

**Reduce your intake of foods high in calories.**

- PROTEINS: handled store meats, tofu, bacon, sausages, and grilled meats.

- Cereal bars, liquids from organic products, honey, molasses, natural products that are canned, dried, and pureed sugar, pop, wafers, pretzels, chips, fries, candies, doughnuts, biscuits, baked goods, and cakes are examples of starches. Note: There are also plenty of fats in these food sources. Understand the substances that are fat and sugar!

- FATS: bacon, sausages (a source of protein but not a less beneficial fat source), spread, margarine with cheddar cheese, canola oil, soybean safflower oil, maize oil, and sunflower oil.

## Measure parts

You can use your hand as a portable measuring device anywhere. This helps you divide even more appropriately.

- One component of protein is your palm.
- A bunch of veggies represents a clenched hand.
- You have a piece of starch in your measured hand.
- The thumb is a fatty portion.

**Falling In Love With Midlife**

**Hold on to your desires.**

Not all food cravings are bad. They are often an indication from your body that there is an imbalance in your chemicals. This is often insulin, which controls your blood sugar. Learn to recognize and regulate your desires.

**Keep a record of the food variety you eat.**

Keeping track of your food sources, whether through a spreadsheet, a graph, or a simple journal, allows you to see any patterns in your eating habits and make the necessary adjustments to improve your energy and overall well-being.

**Possess your alcohol**

When people ask me if I can follow a healthy diet and yet enjoy a glass of wine—or two—I say that I can as long as I remain in control of my choices! Alcohol is a macronutrient that has unique benefits and risks. Given your admittance of six servings of carb packages today—three wines and three beers—I would advise keeping in mind your energy balance for the "EAT LESS" carb class. This helps you match your alcohol consumption to your goals for well-being and health.

**Adopt healthy behaviors to bolster your nutrition strategies.**

If you consume the food sources and flavors, are capable of preparing or cooking the food variety, and find the portion sizes to be acceptable, you may follow a different dietary pattern. Don't make things too complicated. Establish your routine to make food prep simple and your method sustainable.

## What exercise routines are best suited for me in midlife?

Finding the correct workout program in middle age is essential to maintaining general health, energy levels, and true wellness. Our bodies need a balanced approach as we age, which includes high-impact workouts, strength training, flexibility, and balance exercises. This is a detailed guide on the best workout regimens for midlife.

**Energy-dense exercise**

For what purpose does it matter? Exercise with a high impact improves cardiovascular health, increases stamina, and manages weight. It also eases pressure and supports temperament.

*Recommended Activities*:

- Trolling: This low-impact activity ought to be feasible everywhere. For around half an hour, five days a week, don't hold anything back. Strolling can be easily included in your daily schedule and is easy on the joints.

- Riding an exercise bike or riding outside, cycling improves leg strength and cardiovascular health. It's also a low-impact workout that people with joint problems can do.

- Swimming: Provides a full-body workout with very little joint strain. Cardiovascular health, muscle strength, and endurance can all be enhanced by swimming. Water-based heart-pumping fitness programs are also a good option.

- movement: Along with being enjoyable and social, movement improves cardiovascular health, balance, and coordination. Think about taking a dance class or simply dancing at home to your favorite song.

## Strengthening Up

For what purpose does it matter? Strength training maintains mass, increases bone density, aids in digestion, and enhances general strength and adaptability.

*Exercises to Try*:

- Weight training: Use machines, opposition groups, or freeloads. Concentrate on large muscle groups such as the arms, back, legs, and chest. Strive for the gold by enrolling in three strength-training classes per week, interspersed with roughly one day off in between.

- Body-Weight Exercises: You should be able to perform exercises like push-ups, squats, rushes, and boards anywhere and without any special equipment. Through these workouts, balance, and fortitude are further developed.

- Opposition Groups: Small and adaptable, these groups can be used for a variety of exercises targeting different muscle areas. They are particularly useful for subtly increasing opposition.

## Adjustability and Setting Up Equilibrium

For what purpose does it matter? Exercises for balance and adaptability help prevent injuries, maintain mobility, and lower the risk of falls. They can also alleviate chronic pain and help with posture development.

***Exercises to Try:***

- Yoga: Combines breathing techniques, postures, and introspection. Strength, balance, and flexibility are all improved by yoga. It also promotes relaxation and mental clarity. Yoga comes in a variety of forms, from the gentle Hatha to the amazing Vinyasa or Power Yoga.

- Judo: A traditional Chinese military skill involving deliberate, steady advancement and deep relaxation. For more experienced adults in particular, yoga is beneficial as it enhances balance, flexibility, and mental focus.

- Stretching: Make stretching exercises a part of your regular regimen. Concentrate on large muscle groups and hold each stretch for 20 to

30 seconds. It should be feasible to extend independently or following workouts.

## Center Strengthening

For what purpose does it matter? A strong core supports overall body strength, enhances balance and steadiness, and reduces the risk of lower back pain.

*Exercises to Try*:

- Pilates: Emphasizes body shaping, flexibility, and center strength. Pilates movements can be done with special equipment or on a mat.

- Abdominal Exercises: Include movements such as leg rises, crunches, and boards. These exercises target the abs and help develop strength in certain regions.

## Why is high-intensity interval training (HIIT) important?

HIIT consists of brief bursts of intense activity interspersed with rest or low-intensity workouts. It can improve digestive health, increase cardiovascular fitness, and help you burn calories much more quickly.

***Exercises to Try:***

- Timespans: Incorporate running, jumping jacks, or burpees as force exercises. Follow these with rest intervals or low-intensity workouts. With any kind of aerobic exercise, such as cycling, swimming, or running, this ought to be achievable.

- Modified HIIT Courses: HIIT sessions tailored to different degrees of wellness are available at many fitness clubs. These sessions offer structured workouts that can be customized to meet each student's needs.

**Body-Mind Exercises**

For what purpose does it matter? Mind-body exercises combine physical development with relaxation techniques and mental focus. They improve general prosperity, aid in lowering stress, and improve mental clarity.

*Exercises Suggestions:*

- Meditation: Regular meditation can reduce stress, improve health at home, and sharpen attention. Combining contemplation with mild physical work, such as strolling meditation, can provide additional benefits.

- Qigong: A traditional Chinese form of meditation, breathing, and assisted development. Qigong can enhance one's abilities to maintain balance, adjust, and focus.

## How Can I Be Sure I'm Getting Just the Right Amount of Sleep and Recuperation?

Especially as we get older, rest and recuperation are essential components of a healthy lifestyle. Ensuring that you receive the ideal balance between rest and recuperation will improve your overall health, mental well-being, and real performance. Here's a detailed explanation of how to maximize your rest and recuperation.

## Understanding the Importance of Recovery and Rest

Rest and recuperation enable your body to repair and alter tissues, lower the risk of injury, and improve performance. Mental capacity, overall health, and stress reduction are all correlated with mental rest.

## Emphasizing Repose

Getting enough sleep is essential for preserving one's physical and mental well-being. It enables the body to bind memories, repair tissues, and control chemicals.

- Establish a Dependable Rest Schedule: Even on the weekends, dependably go to bed and wake up at the same time. This Regulates the internal clock of your body.

- Create a loosening Sleep schedule: Before going to bed, do some peaceful activities like reading, thinking, or doing the dishes.

- Enhance Your Sleep Environment: Make sure your room is quiet, dark, and cold. Invest in comfortable pillows and a sleeping mat.

- Limit your screen time before night. The production of melatonin, the hormone that regulates sleep, can be slowed down by being open to blue light from screens. At least one hour before going to bed, turn off all electronics.

## Including Rest Days in Your Workout Schedule

Days of rest are crucial for the growth and repair of muscles. Overtraining can result in fatigue, poor performance, and injury.

- Arrange Typical Rest Days: You should incorporate a few days of recuperation into your weekly workout regimen. Use these days to either fully rest or engage in modest activity.

- Keep your body in mind when you stand: Pay attention to signs of overtraining, such as irritated muscles, crankiness, and severe tiredness. Similarly, modify your schedule.

- Initiate Dynamic Recovery: To promote blood flow and recuperation without overtaxing your body on rest days, think about doing low-impact workouts like walking, gentle yoga, or stretching.

## Practicing Unwinding Techniques

For what purpose does it matter? Relaxation techniques can improve brain clarity, decrease heart rate, and reduce tension. Constant pressure can hinder healing and harm health.

- Deep Breathing Exercises: To calm the brain and lower blood pressure, engage in profound breathing exercises. Try techniques like the

4-7-8 breathing technique or diaphragmatic breathing.

- Moderate muscular Relaxation: To apply pressure, this involves tensing and then slowly relaxing different muscular groups.

- caring and Contemplation: Make caring reflection a regular part of your day. This can aid in lowering stress, enhancing profound prosperity, and improving attention.

- Yoga and Kendo: These mind-body exercises combine real-world postures with breathing and relaxation techniques to enhance both mental and physical relaxation.

**Balancing Physical Activity and Rest**

For what purpose does it matter? You can benefit from physical activity without going overboard if you approach it in a balanced manner. Rehabilitation considers improved performance as well as a lower risk of harm.

- Vary Up Your Workouts: Alternate between low-power and intense attention exercises. Include a variety of exercises, such as cardiovascular, strength training, and flexibility exercises.

- Examine Your Strength: Use tools such as saw effort scales or pulse screens to make sure you're not consistently overexerting yourself.

- Combine Portability and Stretching Exercises: These can reduce muscle tension and promote additional adaptation, which will aid in recovery.

## Nutrition and Hydration for Healing

For what purpose does it matter? Sufgestion and hydration are essential for muscle repair, energy replenishment, and overall recovery.

- Drink plenty of water: Throughout the day, especially before, during, and after your workout, sip a lot of water. Dehydration can impair recovery and performance.

- Adopt a Balanced Diet: Make sure you get a variety of carbohydrates, proteins, and good fats. Proteins aid in muscle repair, carbohydrates replenish glycogen stores, and lipids are essential for overall health.

- Post-Exercise Nourishment: Within 30 to 2 hours of working exercise, eat a snack or meal high in carbohydrates and protein. This repairs muscles and replenishes glycogen stores.

## Making Use of Recovery Tools and Techniques

For what purpose does it matter? Recuperation equipment and techniques can improve muscle recovery, reduce sensitivity, and improve overall well-being.

What more can be done?

- Froth Rolling: Using foam rollers for self-myofascial release can help improve healing, increase blood flow, and provide muscle tightness.

- Knead Treatment: Regular back massages help reduce tension in the muscles, promote blood flow, and facilitate relaxation.
- Cold and Force Therapy: Alternating between cold and power treatments can reduce discomfort, ease the sensitivity of the muscles, and accelerate healing.
- Strain Garments: After a workout, wearing strained garments can improve circulation and lessen tense muscles.

**Observing Recoveries and Modifying Schedules**

Why is it important? Recognizing your recuperation aids in determining your body's needs and modifying your daily schedule to prevent injuries and overtraining.

What ought to be genuinely achievable?

- Monitor Your Actions: Maintain a record of your screen power, duration, and repetitions. Take note of any indications of fatigue or unease.
- Employ Devices and Applications for Recovery: Use recovery applications or well-being monitors that monitor rest quality, overall recovery status, and heart rate variability (HRV).

# Chapter Three

## How Might I Oversee and Forestall Midlife crisis?

A midlife crisis is a timeframe during which a singular person feels new or deteriorating pressure and profound uneasiness in life because of their passing youth. The idea arose during the 1960s alongside the thought that individuals arrived at their tops by age 35. Thus, all that came after was a time of decline. One could see their exhibition and generally life turning out to be less alluring, so would hence fall into a midlife crisis. This could last half a month, months, or in additional outrageous cases, years.

## Falling In Love With Midlife

Studies make sense that one's "midlife" is a period connected with low joy and levels of life fulfillment. Psychological wellness experts have additionally distinguished a "U-formed" movement of joy during an individual's life. Joy is most noteworthy during youth, early adulthood, and later adulthood. Many normally experience a satisfaction plunge during midlife, however, this isn't true for everybody.

## Is a Midlife Crisis a Legend?

Midlife emergencies are not a legend, and many experience emergencies through different pieces of their life and achievements ages, not simply in that frame of mind of their life (quarter-life emergencies are likewise normal). Essentially a fourth of grown-ups have encountered a midlife crisis. While a midlife crisis is not a diagnosable condition, the encounters of profound overpower and crisis can be viewed as a component of other psychological well-being state of mind and change problems. A portion of the signs remember changes in weight, rest and dietary patterns, and changes in connections, work, and individual cleanliness.

## <u>Do Women Go Through a Midlife Crisis?</u>

Studies have shown that women are not resistant to going through a midlife crisis, but the experience is particularly unique for a woman than for a man. A midlife crisis for a woman might happen whenever in midlife, with age 40 being the beginning of this formative period.

Women's midlife emergencies, notwithstanding, are much of the time the summit of a large number of co-happening stressors, including well-being or clinical issues, providing care jobs both for youngsters and for maturing guardians, and misfortunes connected with death or separation.

**Falling In Love With Midlife**

**1. Despondency or Expanded Burdensome Ways of behaving**

Midlife for women is a period wherein there can be expanded menopause and sadness, and this time of life is portrayed as having more significant levels of self-destruction contrasted with other life stages.

**2. Reflection On Profound Inquiries or Distraction With Existential Worries**

Due to the obvious existential acknowledgment (i.e., existential emergencies) that somebody has at midlife, a lady might wind up scrutinizing her life decisions like her significant other, profession, or decisions connected with becoming (or not having turned into) a mother.

**3. Rest Issues**

Rest changes connected with perimenopause or menopause can be an indication that a woman is going into the midlife period. A woman reports experiencing issues dozing because of fretfulness or hot blazes.

## 4. Changes In Weight

Weight reduction or weight gain is related with close-to-home changes in individuals. At the point when certain individuals are focused on or going through a crisis, their craving frequently becomes smothered subsequently. Others adapt to close-to-home pressure by working out, which can prompt a weight decline. For some others, they might eat when they are close to home as a method for adapting and view eating as relieving.

## 5. Feeling of Weariness or Unresponsiveness

Maybe it's not sorrow, but rather somebody might wind up with a general sensation of uncertainty in the midlife period which might appear as weariness, disregard, or an absence of inspiration.

## 6. Feeling of Misfortune

During any crisis, there is a fundamental sensation of a deficiency of dependability. It tends to be difficult to recognize why we might be feeling misfortune, yet the deficiency of steadiness and security can truly feature how much a midlife crisis influences us.

## 7. Examining a Major Change

Assuming you end up considering rolling out huge improvements in your own or proficient life, this could be an indication that you are drawing nearer a midlife crisis.

## 8. Focusing On "Ancient times"

A distraction from the encounters you had during your more youthful years or needing to remember encounters intended for different times of your life could demonstrate uneasiness with midlife.

## 9. Want to Change Actual Appearance

Like yearning for earlier long stretches of one's life, a lady in a midlife crisis might end up zeroing in on her appearance and tracking down ways of looking more youthful, either through dress or through rolling out actual improvements to hairdo, taking into account surgeries, or just investigating her demeanor toward rolling out superficial improvements.

## 10. Outrageous Sensations of "Overpower"

However, there are stressors whenever of life, the "bunching" impact of numerous job stressors can add to huge sensations of menopause and nervousness, stress, or overpower ladies in midlife.

## 11. Profound Unpredictability

Changes in capacity to deal with feelings and having feelings that present as serious one second and dull the following could show indications of a midlife crisis in a lady. On the off chance that your already accommodating ways have been supplanted by feeling unstable or excessively handily set off, you might be encountering midlife concerns.

## 12. Actual Agony

Abrupt surprising or unexplained actual torment is an obvious indicator that your body and brain are going through pressure. This can be a midlife crisis or something different, however, actual torment is many times a psychosomatization of close-to-home torment.

## 13. Changes In the Monthly cycle

Indications of perimenopause can happen as soon as the mid-thirties, and 12 back to back a very long time without a period is characteristic of the full change to menopause. These hormonal movements might be an indication that a woman is completely entering the midlife period.

## Reasons for Emotional meltdown In women

Reasons for a midlife crisis in women may be catalyzed by natural changes or by social moves that are bountiful in this time of life, like changes in proficient jobs, expanded providing care liabilities, the passing of a parent, and migration of kids. Numerous ladies experience dejection due to being unsure about their character, or in any event, hitting an achievement birthday and feeling the birthday blues.

**Falling In Love With Midlife**

**A woman may experience a midlife crisis for the following reasons:**

- increased "hybrid stressors" from various occupations
- hormonal alterations related to menopause or perimenopause
- feeling lonely in their partnership or marriage
- Changes in character, such as a personality crisis
- Diminished productivity
- Bemoan not having children
- Relationship issues such as divorce
- A sense of emptiness arises in the family once the last child leaves.
- Deaths of relatives and friends
- Taking care of guardians as they mature
- Taking care of children
- Adult children receive back
- Vocational detachment or apathy
- Concerns about bequeathing an "inheritance"

<u>**Strategies for Women Handling a Midlife Crisis**</u>

While a woman's midlife crisis may be upsetting, it may also be an excellent opportunity to revisit past experiences and engage in introspection as your true adult self. Going through a midlife crisis doesn't have to be a scary experience if you can find new qualities or hobbies or connect with others during this shared time.

**Here are thirteen strategies for women to deal with a midlife crisis:**

*1.  Locate or create a neighborhood*

It is so powerful to be surrounded by other ladies who are experiencing similar things. Attend a meeting at work or organize one in your community to talk about the foundations of being a woman in her middle years. This can help you fight off the depression that so often comes with being a woman in her middle years.

*2.  Start a Journal or Diary*

**Falling In Love With Midlife**

If you're concerned about inheriting something, this is a great time to start recording your life! Not only is keeping a diary a wonderful way to document your emotions, but by writing down your tale, you are also creating your legacy. Possessing a distinctive thing that you may want to gift to loved ones or friends at some point can be both therapeutic and playful.

*3. Exercise*

There's never been a better moment to start or alter your regular exercise routine. Physical activity is a fantastic way to maintain your physical health and establish community. It can also help with sleep disorders associated with menopause and other natural midlife changes. Developing or maintaining healthy habits now might improve your overall physical and domestic well-being.

*4. Examine "Midlife Movement" instead of "Midlife Crisis"*

The term "crisis" has the root "choice point," indicating that there is room to go in several directions. Choose to accept this important stage of life as a springboard into a new era full of exciting potential opportunities.

5. *Permit Your Companion To Follow You*

Even though we often feel alone in our interactions, we occasionally hesitate to talk to others about what we're going through out of a paranoid fear of hurting or upsetting friends and family. However, your partner is most likely going through a similar transition. Embracing them in your emotional state can be a fantastic way to promote stronger relationships. Talk to a trusted friend or relative about your plans if you don't have a partner.

6. *Start Something New and Novel*

This is an excellent chance to learn more about a subject or cross something off your "list of must-dos" when it comes to a class you've always had to take or a trip to a place you've always wanted to go. This will keep your mind active and provide your brain with fresh connections to work with.

*7.  Take Career Guidance Into Account*

If you are experiencing exhaustion or discomfort in your line of work, career counseling might help you manage your thoughts before making a shift in your line of work. Many women in their middle years end up reevaluating the career they first chose, armed with fresh knowledge and self-awareness due to shifts in family presumptions. Speaking with a professional career counselor might help you look at potential next steps.

*8.  Examine Your Characteristics*

Given the existential issues that midlife can bring up, this might be a fantastic opportunity to explore your values and how you're living in things that are important to you. You can make changes to live more in line with your attributes by looking into and identifying the core beliefs you live by.

9. *Establish Communication with a Former Self of Yours*

Many women reach midlife and become empty nesters, unable to adequately care for their children daily. Moving back toward past interests or endeavors can be a powerful step, especially when many women have preserved their hobbies or pastimes during their years of raising children. Locate the things you've neglected and allow them to re-enter your life.

10. *Reestablishing a Connection With Nature is highly healing.* Research suggests that spending 20 minutes a day in nature effectively worsens the negative consequences on mental health. In terms of pressure management, nature is an amazing mediator. It may help you find yourself when you feel lost or insane.

11. *Attend to your physical well-being sincerely*

Beyond the regular workout, midlife can be a great time to participate in a general health evaluation, schedule those routine checkups that have been put offfor a long time, or schedule consultations with specialists in areas where your health may need special attention, such as meeting with a dietitian.

*12. Recognize Books*

Reading can be a fantastic way to prepare for emergencies. You could read diaries or books based on real-world events to get a different perspective on life. It is possible to comprehend fiction and get lost in narratives. To learn more about adjusting to your emotions, you can also read books on psychoeducation and self-improvement.

*13. Consult a Counselor*

Starting therapy might help you deal with all of the changes that are happening in your life. Have a conversation with a trusted friend or partner to learn more about their mental process.

**Falling In Love With Midlife**

**When Do Men Experience a Midlife Crisis?**

Experts acknowledge that males experience midlife crises typically between the ages of 40 and 60.

The preparation for a midlife crisis is largely dependent on one's circumstances rather than their age. When faced with unusual challenges, a 38-year-old is just as likely as a 63-year-old to have a midlife crisis. Similarly, just because someone has deliberately gone through one midlife crisis doesn't mean they won't go through another. It is possible to survive multiple emergencies in middle age.

**Do Midlife Emergencies Occur?**

While midlife emergencies are real, mainstream society may have a very inaccurate perception of their impact and frequency. The concept gained traction and was supported by the media. Investing in sports cars, donning hairpieces, and pursuing romantic relationships with younger women are among the pursuits that have been linked to midlife crises.

Between 10 and 20 percent of people claim to have experienced a midlife crisis. The others experience a somewhat fulfilled adult life as they navigate the center. They experience the U-shaped curve of satisfaction, but it never reaches crisis proportions.

## Eight Signs That a Man Is Having a Midlife Crisis

One of the signs of a midlife crisis could be an unanticipated, emotional shift in mood, habits, and way of life. Conversely, it may represent a growing departure from the newly established norm. Everything depends on the man and the situation.

**Here are eight indicators that a man is having a midlife crisis:**

*1. A decline in life satisfaction*

It could very well be an attempt to notice a shift in another person's sense of contentment in life, but some men may exhibit blatant symptoms, such as complaining more frequently or focusing more of their efforts on complaining. Under such conditions, a man might start speculating negatively, saying things like "life sucks."

Men who experience this kind of disillusionment may start blaming others or themselves for not having opened enough doors in their lives. However, if they take full responsibility, this may exacerbate feelings of guilt, resentment, and disappointment.

*2. Deeper Resentment*

A man's mindset will likely be impacted by a midlife crisis. Some will turn to self-indulgence, disappointment, and bitterness. They may sleep more, eat more, and give up on their goals as they feel uninspired and unfulfilled in life.

*3. Wider Shifts in Temperament*

Men who experience a midlife crisis vary in their sudden and rapid shifts in mental states. They can be completely alone and miserable one day, and the next thing they know, they'll be planning a celebration to share with their loved ones.

*4. Unrestricted Path*

Men often behave impulsively and with incorrect thinking during midlife emergencies. They look at several unfavorable adjusting skills as they desperately try to solve their worries. Without consulting their friends and family, they may begin abusing drugs, drinking alcohol, playing games of chance, or organizing costly vacations.

*5. A Focus on Modification*

A person going through a midlife crisis is primarily concerned with their current state of despair, hence they will seek and seek out change.

***Among the alterations associated with a midlife crisis are:***

- New clothes or cars
- fresh relationships
- fresh workouts
- Changes in profession

- Traveling or relocating

6. *Completing Arrangements or Giving Up*

Men experiencing a midlife crisis may believe that they are no longer able topursue new goals in life. If they think set goals are too difficult or not worth the effort, they may give up on them.

7. *Unhappiness and irritability toward job, family, or oneself*

In a midlife crisis, disappointment, irritability, and outrage are common, especially in men, who tend to express their distress more often than women through outrage. The three things they could concentrate on were themselves, their family, and/or their work.

8. *Being Taken Away*

A man going through a crisis may start to distance himself from people and become detached. They can be too disappointed in themselves for the choices that led to their unhappiness, or they might feel too ashamed of their current situation. Men may also enclose those they have surrounded themselves with to express their discontent, suffering, and disappointment, as they may hold others responsible for their mishandled openings and present lack of fulfillment.

## Stages in Male Midlife Crises

Even while male midlife crises aren't always severe, unlike other situations, there may still be observable signs of one.

**Men may experience a midlife crisis in five stages, which include:**

- **The initial phase:** The individual is in this stage of his usual behavior before the crisis.

- **The crisis's descent:** The descent into the crisis could be moderately protracted or sudden and rapid.

- **The foundation:** The lower phase of the crisis is characterized by heightened adverse effects, a lowered mood, and acute anguish.

- **The move:** Either via their actions or the passage of time, the guy will eventually begin to emerge from the crisis.
- **The new normal**: After the crisis has passed, the man will return to his normal routine.

## What Leads to a Man's Midlife Crisis?

Men's midlife crises can have a variety of causes, depending on the individual, their situation, their support system, and their pressures. An unpleasant situation could lead to a crisis if it occurs at an inappropriate time.

**A male midlife crisis could arise for nine reasons, including:**

1. **Growing up:** Men may struggle to accept who they are becoming in comparison to their former selves as they genuinelyage.
2. **Separate**: Although a big change forces a man to reassess his life and future, separation

can catalyze a midlife crisis; melancholy following a separation is rather common.

3. **Existential concerns**: Where have you been, who are you, and where are you going? These questions have the potential to trigger an existential or midlife crisis.

4. **Children becoming older**: Children's timetables, activities, and daily schedules will no longer dominate life as they leave the house for school or other educational settings. This newly found opportunity can be quite uncomfortable and full of vulnerability; it can sometimes be compared to the empty sensation that remains in the home after the final child leaves.

5. **Work shift or elevation**: People frequently join the workforce with expectations of the improvements and successes they will achieve. However, a lot of jobs don't end that way, or they might reach a certain point in a

person's career. A person who is experiencing a decline in their career or is depressed upon retirement or a job loss may eventually experience a midlife crisis.

6. **Guardians' age progression:** Growing guardians require more thought and attention, which may result in new challenges and routines.

7. **Health worries**: Even a previously healthy guy may have a remarkable health alert as he approaches middle age, forcing him to rearrange his priorities.

8. **loved someone's death:** Events have the power to make men consider their demise as deaths become more frequent or severe. With a midlife crisis, passing is also associated with feelings of sadness and tragedy, as well as discouragement, which can never truly separate from one another.

9. **The triumphs of others:** Men are cunning, thus learning about another man's achievements and successes could make one reflect on their seeming flaws and spiral into a crisis.

## Guidelines for Adjusting to a Midlife Crisis

Although a man doesn't have to take action to seek assistance for the negative consequences of midlife crises, a man will take action to effectively adjust to and lessen their unfavorable outcomes. These can be simple, like recognizing and sharing their ideas with a support group and identifying healthy habits, but they can also include finding qualified aid.

**Here are ten strategies for men to deal with a midlife crisis:**

**1. Recognize Your Feelings**

**Falling In Love With Midlife**

Make sure you conduct a thorough inquiry into your feelings. Pay attention to your feelings and make an effort not to discount or minimize their importance.

## 2. Express Your Thoughts

Share your feelings with people once you've got them under control. Inform your loved ones about your feelings, the reason behind your perception, and how they can support you. You could attempt to benefit from group therapy.

## 3. Make Your Feelings Consistent

Experiencing a midlife crisis is normal. You reject yourself if you reject what is happening. Recognize that midlife crises are completely normal and not exceptional.

## 4. Build Up a Group

Although you may face your issue alone, working through it in a group will help you overcome it. Recruit a supportive network of friends, family, associates, and, rather unexpectedly, your partner.

## 5. Take Another Look at Maturing

**Falling In Love With Midlife**

It's up to you to mature. You might begin to reevaluate how you perceive your development and what lies ahead by shifting your presumptions.

**6. Avoid the Entanglements**.

During a crisis, the impulse to make snap judgments and strong conclusions will be a huge asset. Remain calm and focus on making decisions for the future based on your long-term outcomes rather than your immediate happiness.

**7. Get Your Motivation Back**

A significant portion of the pessimism associated with a crisis stems from uncertainty about one's work and prospects. Spend time with your support group thinking about your motivation and any other goals you may have for your life. Will you continue in the same direction or make a change?

**8. Remain cognizant of Your True Health**

Your mental health will suffer during a midlife crisis, but you still need to take care of your physical health. Prioritize obtaining plenty of exercise, restful sleep, and healthy food. Any issue is hard to face when you're exhausted, sleepy, and hungry.

## 9. Appreciate the Shift

Change is a constant in daily life, but during a midlife crisis, it also causes express concern. Learn to appreciate and accept the new challenges that lie ahead of you rather than dwelling on your fear or anxiety about the change.

## 10. Respect the Journey

Tolerating the path through a midlife crisis may be the best course of action. You will have a remarkably unique midlife experience. Recognize the steps you are taking to control your harmful desires.

## How can I continue to be proactive in getting regular health screenings?

Maintaining optimal health and affluence in midlife requires being vigilant about routine health checks.

**Falling In Love With Midlife**

Our risk of developing certain health disorders increases with age, which makes early detection through screenings much more fundamental.

Here are some steps to help you continue to be proactive in your midlife years regarding routine health screenings:

***Recognize the Importance of Health Screenings in Midlife***

Midlife represents a transition into an age where some health risks become more prevalent, making it a crucial time for health exams. Knowing the importance of these tests will encourage you to prioritize them in your healthcare plan. Regular screenings can detect diseases that take into account early intervention and treatment, such as diabetes, hypertension, cholesterol, colorectal illness, bosom malignant growth, and prostate malignant growth, among others.

## *Be Aware of the Screenings You Should Do*

Rules about health screenings are determined by various health associations based on variables such as family history, age, sexual orientation, and other risk factors. Learn about the screenings that are advised for individuals in their middle years and discuss them with your healthcare provider. In midlife, standard screenings could include bone thickness testing, mammograms, Pap smears, colonoscopies, prostate exams, cholesterol checks, and circulatory strain monitoring.

## *Arrange Routine Inspections*

Make time to schedule routine examinations with your primary care physician or other healthcare provider. During these consultations, you can discuss your overall health, address any side effects or concerns, and choose which exams are appropriate for you based on your unique health profile and risk factors. Don't withhold anything from the real assessment to ensure that your health needs are met consistently.

### *Establish Follow-Up and Updates*

Set reminders for upcoming screenings and appointments to capitalize on your innovative side. You may arrange changes well in advance with many schedule programs, which ensures you remember to make or show up for your appointments. To ensure congruency of care, make sure to promptly follow up with your healthcare provider regarding any unexpected results or suggested follow-up tests or treatments.

### *Continue to Communicate Openly with Your Healthcare Provider*

Maintaining a proactive approach to your health checks requires establishing a trusting connection with your healthcare provider. Take proactive steps to investigate any concerns or side effects you may be experiencing, as well as any medical history of illnesses or disorders in your family. Your healthcare provider can provide tailored screening and preventive estimate suggestions based on your unique health profile.

### *Emphasis on Health Prevention*

In addition to routine tests, focus on preventative health actions to reduce your risk of developing chronic illnesses and diseases. This includes adopting a healthy lifestyle, maintaining a regular eating schedule, engaging in regular physical labor, managing stress, obtaining enough sleep, and abstaining from tobacco and excessive alcohol use. These lifestyle choices can enhance general prosperity and serve as a supplement to routine screenings.

### *Continue to learn and be a self-supporter*

Keep up with the latest guidelines about midlife health screening recommendations and preventive measures. Speak up for yourself by asking questions, seeking clarification, and insisting on examinations or tests that you believe are essential to your well-being. Remember that when it comes to your success and well-being, you are the best advocate for yourself.

***Incorporate Your Supportive Network Emotionally***

Inform your loved ones, friends, or network of people who can provide emotional support about your health goals and needs. They can offer support throughout exams or treatments, offer encouragement, and assist you in remembering upcoming appointments. Being proactive about health checks doesn't have to feel burdensome; rather, it can seem more rational when one has an emotionally supporting network.

## What lifestyle changes can help me manage or prevent chronic conditions?

Examining midlife offers an opportunity to reevaluate and improve your lifestyle choices to promote long-term health and wealth. Through proactive lifestyle changes, you can effectively manage or prevent the ongoing situations that are typically associated with this stage of life. Here are several significant lifestyle adjustments that have been specially designed for midlife and can help you stay active and healthy:

1. Establish a heart-healthy diet by emphasizing whole grains, organic produce, lean meats, and healthy fats

- Limit managed high-sodium items, processed carbs, and a variety of foods.
- Screen segment sizes to support heart health and the board's weight.

2. Maintain Physical Dynamism: Engage in regular high-impact exercise, weight training, and activities that enhance flexibility and balance.

- Choose workouts that you enjoy and can stick with over time to help practicing become a regular part of your day.

3. Effectively Manage Pressure:

- Employ relaxation techniques such as deep breathing, introspection, or gentle muscle relaxation.
- To prevent feeling overwhelmed, concentrate on self-care activities and record realistic presumptions and stopping points.

4. Put Quality Rest First:

- Create a more flexible sleep schedule and maintain a consistent rest strategy.
- Make sure your sleeping environment promotes restful sleep and minimizes screen time before bedtime.

5. Maintain a Healthy Weight: To prevent overindulging, eat mindfully and monitor portion sizes.

- Include regular, physically demanding work in your everyday routine to assist in balancing the executives.

# <u>EMOTIONAL LIFE</u>

# Chapter Four

## What can Enhanced Emotional Intelligence Do for Me?

Gaining more emotional intelligence may be a very helpful tool, especially when learning about the complexities and challenges of midlife. Here's how gaining emotional intelligence can significantly impact your life at this point:

**Worked on Mindfulness:** Enhanced emotional intelligence enables you to cultivate a deeper understanding of your own emotions, strengths, weaknesses, and values. Being aware becomes more important in midlife since you may experience big life-altering experiences and advancements. Understanding your emotions and their underlying causes will help you make better decisions that are consistent with your goals and moral principles. By practicing mindfulness, you can investigate midlife with confidence and legitimacy, leading to the development of a stronger sense of fulfillment and logic.

**Increased Pressure The board:** Midlife is often accompanied by increased responsibilities, conflicts, and strains; these can range from issues with one's career to obligations to one's family to worries about one's health. Enhanced emotional intelligence gives you the tools to effectively manage pressure through emotional regulation, self-care practice, and seeking assistance when needed. You can explore midlife advancements with ease and elegance by developing strength and survival skills, which will lessen the negative impact of weight on your overall prosperity.

**Better Connections:** Whether it's fostering new kinships, extending cherished ties, or investigating deep connections, midlife is the time when connections become even more significant. Improved emotional intelligence gives you the ability to make more meaningful connections by strengthening your capacity for empathy, communication, and compromise. Understanding and sensitivity to the emotions of others allows you to strengthen relationships, constructively resolve conflicts, and build new relationships based on mutual respect, trust, and understanding.

**Expanded Sympathy:** As you become older, developing empathy becomes increasingly important for investigating various social collaborations and identifying opposing viewpoints. Enhanced emotional intelligence enables you to empathize with the experiences and emotions of others, fostering more meaningful empathy and connection. In middle age, empathy can be particularly valuable for filling in generational gaps, mentoring younger partners, and helping guardians as they mature. You may practice compassion and build stronger, more meaningful relationships both naturally and skillfully.

**Better Direction:** Changing careers, planning for retirement, or pursuing new interests are just a few examples of the crucial decisions that characterize midlife. Improved emotional knowledge integrates both rational analysis and emotional experiences to enhance your critical thinking abilities. You can pursue choices that align with your strengths, needs, and long-term goals by considering the emotional consequences of your choices. This comprehensive approach to direction gives you the ability to examine midlife transitions with greater significance, validity, and clarity.

**Improved Versatility:** Midlife can bring its fair share of disasters, discontents, and challenges, ranging from marital problems to career setbacks to concerns about one's health. Improved emotional intelligence promotes adaptability by helping you emerge from adversity with greater resilience and strength. Rethinking challenges as opportunities for growth, learning, and self-discovery will help you become more adaptable and overcome obstacles with assurance, hope, and variety. This adaptability gives you the ability to welcome midlife transitions as opportunities for self-discovery and self-reconciliation rather than as sources of fear or weakness.

**More Notable Affluence:** Lastly, enhanced emotional intelligence contributes to a generally more notable sense of affluence and midlife fulfillment. Through cultivating mindfulness, effectively managing stress, maintaining relationships, and making decisions that are consistent with your values, you can experience a deeper sense of fulfillment, logic, and joy. By concentrating on emotional intelligence in middle age, you can learn to live in the moment, cultivate gratitude, and savor the luxury of life's experiences. You can encounter midlife with more noticeable versatility, credibility, and euphoria by investing in your emotional awareness, which will make it a meaningful and fulfilling aspect of your life process.

## How can I use real-world examples to help me grow emotionally?

Exploring the complexities of midlife and developing more notable strength, shrewdness, and satisfaction can be achieved by using real examples for emotional development. When you reflect on your past experiences and learn from them, you can harness the knowledge you've gained to promote personal development and enhance your emotional well-being. You can use life examples in the following ways to support emotional growth in midlife:

**Reflect on Past Experiences:** Take time to consider important events, relationships, and challenges from a considerable amount of time ago. Think about the lessons learned from these experiences, the two successes and the two setbacks. Thinking back on your history gives you clarity, insight, and understanding of your behavior patterns, worldviews, and emotional responses.

**Separate Important Topics and Illustrations:** Look for everyday topics and instances that come from your experience. These subjects may recall adaptability as the essence of suffering, the value of relationships and associations, or the need for diligence and confidence. You can gain a deeper understanding of your traits, requirements, and areas for growth by identifying recurring patterns.

**Develop Self-Empathy:** Turn to your prior experiences of self-empathy and giving; remember that you are human and prone to error. Accept your flaws and mistakes as opportunities for growth and learning rather than sources of shame or regret. You may maintain a healthy and consistent relationship with yourself, which is essential for emotional development, by learning to empathize with yourself.

**Extract meaning and Intelligence:** Take your life experiences and extract intelligence and meaning by asking yourself questions like,

- What did this experience teach me?
- In what ways has this event shaped my beliefs and principles?
- What traits and attributes have I developed as a result of this experience?
- How can I use the examples to investigate present challenges and create opportunities?

**Falling In Love With Midlife**

Through astute and skillful analysis of your past, you can uncover significant events that contribute to your emotional growth and adaptability.

**Foster Appreciation:** Work on showing gratitude for the lessons you've learned and the growth you've experienced as a result of your interactions. Acknowledge and cherish the people, events, and circumstances that have shaped who you are now. Gaining appreciation promotes an optimistic viewpoint and attitude, which is essential for emotional growth and prosperity.

**Accept Variation and Change:** The middle years are frequently a time of great advancement and change, ranging from shifts in career paths to purging and settling to genuine modifications brought on by growing. Accept these advancements as any kind of opportunity for growth and transformation rather than sources of fear or resistance. Utilize your flexibility and astuteness from past experiences to your advantage as you explore life's interesting turns in the path.

**Establish Development Goals:** Establish development goals for your emotional growth, focusing on areas where you want to increase your mindfulness, adaptability, and believability. Whether it's improving self-control, expanding relationships, or strengthening interpersonal skills, set clear goals and take concrete steps to support your personal growth.

**Seek Assistance and Companionship:** Seek assistance and companionship from individuals who can provide guidance, perspectives, and encouragement during your journey of emotional growth. This could be friends, family, mentors, or experts who can offer valuable information and a firm listening ear. Making contact with others who have experienced similar things can also help one feel accepted and like they belong.

# Falling In Love With Midlife

**Practice Presence and Care:** Focus on the present moment with openness, curiosity, and acknowledgment as you cultivate presence and care in your daily life. You can acquire more notable awareness, emotional control, and strength by engaging in care activities like introspection, deep breathing, or deliberate growth. By settling in today, you may cultivate a sense of clarity and serenity throughout both the good and bad periods of your life.

**Notice Progress and Development:** Acknowledge your progress and development along the way, acknowledging the conclusions you've reached on your journey of emotional growth. Acknowledging your progress encourages constructive adjustments and fosters a strong, confident sense of self. Remember that emotional growth is a long-term process, and every accomplishment is a cause for celebration.

# What steps can I take to cultivate deeper emotional connections?

Gaining more emotional ties in midlife is essential to fostering meaningful connections, improving wealth, and pursuing life's endeavors with greater support and vigor. During this stage of life, you can do the following actions to create new emotional associations:

1. **Get in shape Undivided attention:** Encourage the habit of giving them your whole attention when you communicate with them. Pay close attention to the person speaking, stay in touch, summarize what they've said, and express empathy and understanding by reflecting on their feelings. By demonstrating gratitude, affirmation, and genuine interest in the experiences and

emotions of the other person, undivided attention fosters more connections.

2. **Share Weakness:** Be honest and open with the individuals you trust about your thoughts, feelings, and vulnerabilities. Weakness and credibility are essential components for building emotional bonds because they promote mutual understanding, closeness, and trust. Show who you are and be honest about how you feel, even if it makes you uncomfortable at first.

3. **Develop Compassion:** Put yourself in other people's shoes and attempt to understand their experiences, feelings, and points of view to develop empathy. In addition to recognizing and acknowledging the emotions of others, empathy also entails responding to them with support and understanding. By feeling empathy for other people, you can create

more connections based on our shared humanity and understanding.

4.  **Show Appreciation:** Express gratitude to the people in your life and the meaningful relationships you have with them. Recognizing the value and importance of individuals in your life, appreciation fosters associations, warmth, and appreciation in relationships. Leave time to express gratitude with heartfelt words, acts of kindness, or administrative displays that show how much you value the people in your life.

5.  **Build Trust:** Build trust in your relationships by being trustworthy, consistent, and righteous in your dealings with other people. Deep emotional connections are based on trust because they create a sense of reliability, safety, and security in interpersonal relationships. To foster trust with others, be sincere and direct in your correspondence,

fulfill your obligations, and act honestly in your actions.

6. **Create Shared Encounters:** Create opportunities for meaningful connections and shared experiences with others. common experiences create memories that last a lifetime, whether it's engaging in common hobbies, discovering new interests together, or simply devoting quality time to each other's company. Find activities that you enjoy doing and that help you connect with people more deeply and emotionally.

7. **Put an emphasis on Quality Time:** Allocate a short period for meaningful collaborations and spending time with loved ones. It's critical to prioritize connections and set aside time for association even amid busy schedules and responsibilities. Whether it's scheduling regular family dinners, planning romantic dates, or reaching out to pals for

meaningful conversations, concentrate on creating meaningful opportunities to uphold emotional connections.

8. **Practice Pardoning:** Let go of grudges and grievances from the past to foster empathy and forgiveness in your relationships. For emotional traumas to heal and be fixed, forgiveness is essential because it allows for growth, understanding, and compromise. Accept yourself and others with forgiveness, understanding that we are all fallible and deserving of compassion.

9. **Be Careful and Available:** When working with others, exercise caution and availability while maintaining whole focus and absence of interruptions. By promoting profound tuning in, compassion, and appreciation for the present moment, care enhances emotional linkages. Take care of each other in your daily interactions, enjoy the richness of each moment, and form new relationships with those around you.

# Chapter five

## <u>How Can I Make My Friendships and Family Relationships Stronger?</u>

As I go through midlife, I discover that people are much more aware of the importance of having strong relationships with friends and family. This stage of life often leads to introspection and a deeper respect for those who help and enhance our lives. Building these connections is a functional, conscious effort rather than just a passive happenstance. This is how I try to improve and prepare my relationships with family and friends at this stage of life.

I find that spending quality time with my partners is one of the most effective strategies to build stronger connections. Midlife is a time when it's easy to let personal relationships go to the sidelines due to the demands of work, health issues, raising children, and possibly managing aging parents. I purposefully set aside time for my friends and family to combat this. This may be planning end-of-week get-togethers with friends to escape the daily grind and enjoy each other's company, or it could mean having regular family meals where we can all sit down and share our days. Maintaining strong ties and creating fresh, priceless memories depend on these fellowship photos.

Strong communication is still the cornerstone of healthy relationships, and as I've become older, I've learned to value it much more. Conversations with friends and family can get deeper and more meaningful when one reaches middle age. I place a strong emphasis on being open and honest, offering my thoughts, feelings, and experiences while also acting as a critical observer. When I listen properly, I can better understand my friends and family and respond to them with support and sympathy. It also demonstrates my caring for them. This two-way communication channel promotes mutual respect and trust.

Relationships can be strengthened to a great extent by expressing gratitude. I have a habit of saying thank you, whether it's with a simple "thank you" for a small but kind deed or acknowledging the ongoing support I receive from my friends and family. Acknowledging successes, no matter how small, increases the value I place on our connections. By expressing my gratitude, I let my loved ones know how much they mean to me and how much their presence improves my life.

Understanding and sympathy are important, especially as we all experience distinct midlife struggles and transitions. I try to be understanding, trying to put myself in my friends and family's shoes and understand their struggles. This means that when things get tough, you should be understanding and nonjudgmental while also providing support and comfort when needed. I contribute to the development of trust and resilience by providing emotional support to my family and friends.

Interactions that are shared are yet another effective way to build stronger bonds. I successfully look for opportunities to get us involved in activities that we enjoy as a group. This might be traveling on a journey together, picking up a new hobby, visiting distant developments, or even just watching movies at home regularly. These everyday activities foster a sense of camaraderie and pranks, building a reservoir of positive memories that we can all access. What often binds us together are our shared giggles, projects, and, strangely, failures.

Availability and stability at pivotal moments are essential for building stronger bonds in partnerships. Many challenges might arise in midlife, such as health issues, career shifts, or duties to family members. I make it a point to be there for my friends and family, lending a sympathetic ear or some common sense support when needed. Sometimes, the simple knowledge that someone is supporting you can have a profound impact. I develop the duties of trust and dependability in my relationships by being a consistent source of support.

Maintaining healthy relationships also requires respecting boundaries. Respecting each person's personal space and boundaries is important. I swear that I respect my friend's and family's boundaries and don't impose my boundaries or meddle in their personal space. This mutual respect helps to preserve balance and ensures that our relationships are stable and enduring.

Finally, developing self-awareness and mindfulness becomes essential to preserving partnerships. As I strive to become a better version of myself, I approach my collaborations with people in a more assured and grown-up manner. I can contribute to more fulfilling relationships by being more understanding, tenacious, and emotionally astute. Self-improvement also means identifying and overcoming any internal problems that might be impeding my relationships, such as communication boundaries or unresolved conflicts.

## What can I do to deepen my bonds with loved ones?

Developing bonds with friends and family during midlife requires deliberateness, reflection, and significant activities. The following are a few techniques that can assist with reinforcing these fundamental associations:

**Focus on Quality Time**

- ***Deliberate Commitment:*** amidst occupied plans and various obligations, put forth a cognizant attempt to cut out quality time for loved ones. This could include setting up normal family meals, arranging end-of-the-week excursions, or going through a night together without interruptions. The key is to be available and completely drawn in during these times.

## Cultivate Open Correspondence

- *Fair Discussions:* Correspondence is the groundwork of any solid relationship. Make a place of refuge for transparent discussions. Share your considerations, sentiments, and encounters while empowering your friends and family to do likewise. This common sharing forms trust and understanding.

- *Undivided attention*: Practice undivided attention by really focusing when somebody is talking, showing compassion, and answering nicely. This exhibits regard as well as assists in seeing each other's viewpoints with bettering.

## Show Appreciation and Appreciation

- ***Offer Thanks:*** Consistently express your appreciation for the easily overlooked details your friends and family do. A straightforward "much obliged" or a sincere commendation can have a huge effect. Recognizing their endeavors and offering thanks fortifies the profound association.

- ***Observe Accomplishments:*** Perceive and celebrate both of all shapes and sizes achievements in their lives. Whether it's an advancement work or an individual accomplishment, commending these minutes together cultivates a feeling of shared bliss and pride.

Falling In Love With Midlife

**Fabricate Compassion and Understanding**

- ***Practice Sympathy:*** Try to comprehend and understand the encounters and feelings of your friends and family. Come at the situation from their perspective and attempt to see things according to their viewpoint. This can help in settling clashes and extending profound bonds.

- ***Support During Difficult stretches:*** Show up for your friends and family during testing times. Offer daily reassurance, reasonable assistance, or a listening ear. Your presence and support can give gigantic solace and fortify your relationship.

**Make Shared Encounters**

- ***Participate in Exercises Together:*** Track down exercises and leisure activities that you can partake in together. Whether it's voyaging, cooking, playing sports, or going to far-reaching developments, shared encounters make enduring recollections and reinforce bonds.

- ***Customary Practices:*** Lay out normal customs or ceremonies, for example, a month-to-month game evening or a yearly vacation. These practices give something to anticipate and assist with keeping major areas of strength for an association.

## Regard Limits

- ***Honor Individual Space:*** Everybody needs private reality to themselves. These limits are pivotal for sound relationships. Guarantee that you give your friends and family the space they need without forcing your assumptions on them.

## Center around Self-awareness

- ***Personal growth:*** Work on self-awareness and mindfulness. By turning out to be more quiet, understanding, and sincerely experienced, you can bring a more sure and steady presence into your relationships.

- ***Address Private Matters:*** Perceive and resolve any private matters that may be influencing your relationships, like correspondence boundaries or unsettled clashes.

By carrying out these systems, you can extend your bonds with friends and family, making more grounded, additional satisfying relationships that give bliss, support, and a feeling of having a place during midlife.

# How could I possibly make meaningful new friendships at any point?

Creating new, meaningful friendships in middle age may be rewarding and challenging at the same time. Significant advancements are often seen throughout this stage of life, such as changing careers, navigating complex relationships, and developing self-awareness, all of which can pave the way for meaningful, long-lasting relationships with new people. Here are some tools to help you make meaningful new friendships in your middle years:

## Engage in physical activity and leisure pursuits

Join Clubs and Groups: Take part in physical activities and hobbies that you find enjoyable. A great way to meet others who share your interests is to join clubs, sports teams, or groups related to your hobby. Shared interests provide a solid foundation for new connections, whether they are formed in a reading club, gardening group, or wellness class.

Enroll in Classes: Choose classes or studios based on your interests or professional goals. This creates an environment in which you may interact with people who have similar interests and values and also gives you the chance to learn something new.

## Participate Locally and Volunteer

- *Volunteer Work:* Participate in community service initiatives or volunteer work. Following a common goal fosters a sense of fraternity and provides ample opportunities to network. Additionally, lending a helping hand often attracts kind and well-liked locals who can become amazing friends.

- *Go to Nearby Events:* Participate in community events such as festivals, business gatherings for ranchers or large-scale initiatives to show your support for the community. These get-togethers are perfect for making new friends and striking up conversations in a relaxed setting.

## Impact Expert and Social Organizations

- ***Reconnect with Old Acquaintances:*** Reaching out to former partners, coworkers, or lifelong friends might help to rekindle old friendships and even forge new ones. Social media platforms such as Facebook and LinkedIn are useful tools for reestablishing contact with people you may have lost touch with years ago.

- ***Visit the Events for Systems Administration:*** Participate in industry meetups, events, or activities centered around professional systems administration. These events offer opportunities to network with new people in your professional network, some of whom may end up becoming friends outside of the workplace.

## Be Friendly and Open-Minded

- ***Exhibit Verifiable Interest:*** Take an authentic interest in the lives and interactions of those you meet. Ask open-ended questions and pay close attention to their responses. This demonstrates that you value their opinion and are eager to establish a meaningful relationship.

- ***Be Yourself:*** Establishing verifiable friendships requires credibility. Be authentic and let your true self come out. True connections will inevitably lead to long-lasting connections.

**Falling In Love With Midlife**

**Take a stab at it.**

- *Welcome Individuals Out:* Don't be afraid to take risks when making arrangements. Invite new coworkers to a get-together, stroll, or espresso. Taking the initiative demonstrates your want to understand them better and facilitates the transition from associate to friend.

- *Continue*: After you've met someone else, follow up with a message or phone call to let them know you were happy to meet them and might want to stay in touch. Reliable communication helps establish and maintain new friendships.

**Remain persistent and patient.**

- *Give It Time:* It takes work and dedication to forge meaningful friendships. Have patience and let relationships develop organically. It's important to avoid rushing the conversation or making irrational assumptions.

- *Have Persistence:* If you don't find your new best friend right away, don't give up at all. Keep putting yourself out there, engaging in physical activity, and making new friends. Forging durable relationships requires determination.

## Be Reliable and Firm.

- *Offer Support:* Be a solid and trustworthy friend. When needed, provide support and encouragement, and be present to acknowledge victories and accomplishments. Reliability and support are essential elements of strong friendships.

- *Be Open and Trusting:* True friendships are built on vulnerability and trust. Tell your new friends about your experiences, feelings, and challenges, and encourage them to do the same. By doing this, the association grows and mutual understanding is fostered.

## Apply Creativity

- ***Online Communities:*** Participate in online groups or forums that align with your interests. These online communities can be a fantastic way to meet new people and perhaps turn these online collaborations into real friendships.

- ***Social Media:*** Make use of online entertainment to stay in touch with new coworkers. Maintaining budding connections can be facilitated by exchanging updates, engaging in conversations, and setting up get-togethers via virtual entertainment platforms.

# Chapter Six

## I've learned How to Rekindle Love and Romance in Midlife?

Rekindling romantic feelings in middle age can be a remarkable and beneficial journey. Significant life changes often occur during this time, such as children leaving the house, career changes, or self-awareness, which can have an impact on genuine relationships. However, these steps also offer opportunities to rekindle passion and strengthen your relationship with your partner. I've discovered how to rekindle love and sentiment in my middle years by doing this.

**Prioritize Spending Quality Time Together.**

One of the simplest steps you can take to revive your relationship is to make time for your partner.

## Falling In Love With Midlife

It's easy for the relationship to become secondary as life picks up with duties to family, career, and other pursuits. In response, my partner and I have made a conscious effort to spare each other standard time. We schedule date nights where we can focus solely on one other without any distractions, week after week. Simple dinners at home, walks in the park, or watching movies together can all have a big impact on these dates. They don't have to be extravagant. It is necessary to have the key on hand and pulled in throughout these minutes.

## Convey Transparently and Truly

Strong communication is the foundation of any person's main areas of strength. Over time, I've come to realize how important it is to be open and honest with my partner about my feelings, desires, and worries. We've created a haven where we can talk about anything without worrying about being

# Falling In Love With Midlife

judged. Our ability to be transparent has allowed us to successfully and promptly address any problems or mistakes. We also emphasize listening well to one another and expressing empathy and comprehension. We have been able to reconnect on a deeper level because of this two-way communication channel.

## Re-discover each other

It's easy to slip into routines and habits throughout midlife, which can make a relationship feel stagnant. My accomplice and I have attempted to rediscover each other in an attempt to reignite the flash. We ask each other questions about our goals, interests, and desires, much like we did when we first started dating. This has led to several thought-provoking and poignant conversations. We also explore new hobbies and activities together, which gives our relationship a sense of adventure and vitality.

**Falling In Love With Midlife**

Whether it's attending a culinary class, making a journey to new areas, or analyzing another game, these shared experiences have drawn us closer.

**Express gratitude and love**

Maintaining feelings in a relationship requires communicating love and gratitude. I've learned how to regularly notice and appreciate the little things that my partner often overlooks. Simple expressions of gratitude, heartfelt compliments, or small acts of kindness can make them feel valued and cherished. We also make an effort to demonstrate genuine affection by holding hands, giving hugs, and kissing. These small acts of intimacy contribute to the development of our strong bond and sustain the feeling.

# Falling In Love With Midlife

## Maintain the Sentiment

We have accepted the relevance of suddenness and shock to maintain the feeling. You may add a spark to your relationship by planning unexpected dates, writing each other heartfelt messages, or surprising each other with small gifts. We also reflect on our early days together, going over tender memories and experiences that led to our maddening infatuation. This nostalgia often brings back our shared feelings of warmth and affection.

## Develop Your Self-Awareness

Reviving sentiment requires self-improvement and personal development. I may enter the relationship with more assurance and maturity if I focus on becoming my best self. This means continuing to erode my ability to truly value others, being persistent, and being understanding. When

# Falling In Love With Midlife

both partners are committed to bettering themselves, the overall quality of the relationship is enhanced.

## Seek Expert Guidance as required.

Now and then, even with our best efforts, restoring emotion can be difficult. Seeking expert guidance can be helpful in certain situations. Couples counseling or therapy can provide valuable insights and tools for resolving relationship problems. Working with a specialist has helped my partner and I see each other more clearly and develop better communication strategies.

## Accept Development and Change Together

Significant changes are often achieved in midlife, both individually and in pairs. Maintaining substantial areas of strength for a caring relationship requires embracing these progressions and coming to terms with one another. We now know how to support one another's personal growth and adapt to the changing dynamics of our partnership. This mutual assistance and adaptability have strengthened our ties and maintained our positive relationship.

## How might I go about navigating relationships and love at any point?

Investigating relationships and love in middle age can be rewarding and challenging. This period often brings about significant life changes and fresh perspectives, necessitating deliberate effort to maintain and strengthen meaningful relationships. The following stages can help you explore relationships and love productively during midlife:

### 1. Put Communication First

*Transparent Exchanges:* Continue to communicate openly and honestly with your partner. Express your thoughts, feelings, and worries honestly, and encourage your partner to do the same. This fosters mutual respect and trust, two things that are essential for a healthy partnership.

Practice undivided attention by focusing solely on your partner during their conversation. Condemn them and acknowledge their feelings; this will assist in resolving conflicts and strengthen your relationship.

## 2. Pay Attention to Your Partnership

*Standard Date Nights*: Set up regular date nights to rekindle your relationship and enjoy each other's company without distractions. These moments help to maintain intimacy and enjoyment in the relationship, whether you're eating out, taking a walk, or engaging in a shared hobby.

*Quality Time*: Prioritize quality time above quantity. Engage in activities that bring you closer together and that you both enjoy, such as going on trips, cooking together, or simply having meaningful conversations.

## 3. Express gratitude and affection

*Give Thanks*: Always let your partner know how much you value them. Acknowledge their efforts and express gratitude for both the small and large things they do. This strengthens your closeness and encourages positive feelings.

*Real Warmth*: Maintain physical proximity with handshakes, hugs, and kisses. Touching someone in person is a powerful way to express and maintain affection.

## 4. Adapt to Modifications and Welcome Progress

*Encourage One Another's Development:* Encouraging one another's growth and development. Encourage and support your partner's goals and advantages, and grow and adapt together as you both grow apart.

*Adaptability and Versatility:* Be open to the changes that come with reaching midlife, whether they have to do with career, well-being, or unique dynamics in relationships. Accept these developments as opportunities to strengthen and get closer to your partner.

## 5. Stay up to date on Freedom

*Personal Interests*: While getting to know one another is important, it's as critical to maintain your own benefits and recreational pursuits. Personal fulfillment enhances your wealth and infuses fresh vitality into the partnership.

Set and abide by established boundaries when it comes to sound. Make sure you and your partner

# Falling In Love With Midlife

have the life necessary for personal contemplation and renewal.

## 6. Handle Conflicts Effectively

*Deal with problems as soon as possible*: Don't let minor problems fester. Handle conflicts and false presumptions calmly and quickly. This prevents contempt and facilitates reaching agreements as a group.

*Search for Group Arrangements*: Approach conflicts as a group, focusing on locating frequently profitable agreements. This collaborative approach strengthens your relationship and ensures that you both feel valued and respected.

## 7. Rekindle Emotion

*Maintain the Flash:* Make an effort to maintain the feeling. Arrange surprises, go on free dates, and reflect on your early days together. These activities support maintaining the relationship's ardor and excitement.

*Participate in fresh and communal interactions*: Whether it's exploring new locations, testing out new activities, or learning something new and helpful together, these shared endeavors create enduring memories and strengthen your relationship.

## 8. Seek Skilled Support when Required

*Couples Therapy*: If you're having trouble moving forward or feel trapped, go ahead and get professional help. Couples therapy can provide valuable insights and tools to enhance your relationship and help you work through conflicts.

*Individual Treatment*: Occasionally, personal issues may have an impact on your partnership. You can resolve these challenges and improve your relationship and self-awareness with the help of individual therapy.

## 9. Create a Happy Environment

*Positive Corporations*: Emphasize creating a stable and upbeat environment in your partnership. Honor one another's victories, extend forgiveness, and make an effort to spend happy moments together.

*Shared Vision and Objectives*: Discuss and make adjustments to your shared vision and goals for the future. Making progress toward common goals promotes a sense of rationality and organization in your partnership.

## 10. Don't Give Up

*Mutual obligation*: Maintain significant areas of strength for both your partnership and each other. Recognize that pursuing relationships and love calls for constant effort, perseverance, and dedication.

**Falling In Love With Midlife**

Extended distance Keep in mind a well-developed point of view. Recognize that relationships have phases and that, with mutual effort and accountability, midlife challenges may be successfully managed.

### How can I establish and maintain romantic relationships?

To explore love and relationships in midlife, one must combine intentional effort, flexibility, and self-disclosure. At this point, the complexity of life's experiences often molds a more elaborate, more sophisticated approach to handling emotion. First and foremost, communication ends up being far more important. Maintaining open communication with your spouse enables you to recognize one other's evolving needs and viewpoints. This means practicing your full attention span as well as speaking your truth. Intensely concentrating, expressing empathy, and endorsing your partner's feelings promote a strong close-to-home bond.

Spending quality time together is also essential. Making time for each other in the middle of busy schedules and responsibilities is essential. Regular date nights or activities that you both participate in, no matter how simple or complex, help to maintain the relationship strong.

Engaging in activities that both partners like strengthens the relationship and creates lifelong memories. Warmth and gratitude play important roles in preserving the feeling. Good feelings accumulate when you express gratitude for your partner's efforts regularly and display physical affection by holding hands or giving hugs. Relationships are bonded by these tiny, heartfelt acts of love and thoughtfulness, especially during difficult times.

## Falling In Love With Midlife

Being adaptable is important because midlife usually brings about considerable changes. Encouraging one another's growth and self-awareness can strengthen the bond. Whether it's a career shift, a side hobby, or self-awareness goals, accepting these advancements together fosters mutual respect and strengthens the bond. Maintaining a sense of independence in the partnership is also beneficial. Pursuing personal hobbies and interests brings fulfillment to the relationship and infuses it with fresh vitality. Firm boundaries ensure that each of the two spouses has the personal space needed for introspection and rejuvenation.

Compromise is yet another fundamental area. Getting problems resolved quickly and effectively prevents hatred from growing. Enhancing the sense of cooperation is tackling conflicts together and concentrating on coming up with solutions. The two parties will feel valued and respected thanks to this collaborative approach. Feeling sentimental again often needs a pinch of immediacy. Maintaining an exciting relationship can be achieved by planning shocks, remembering early times together, or even just trying out challenging new activities. Experiences that are shared, like seeing new places or learning something new and helpful, create enduring memories and strengthen the relationship.

Searching for knowledgeable help occasionally can be beneficial. Couples counseling or therapy provides tools and experiences to enhance relationship components and settle conflicts. This can be especially helpful when facing specific problems or significant life transitions. It's crucial to create a favorable environment in the partnership. The connection is strengthened by acknowledging each other's victories, extending grace, and attempting to spend happy moments together. Examining and modifying common goals and aspirations for the future promotes a sense of cooperation and logic.

# Mental life

# Chapter seven

## How I Maintain Mental Health and Clarity?

Maintaining mental clarity and wellness in middle age is a complex endeavor that calls for a variety of approaches. Here's how I thoroughly and in-depth examine this terrain:

- **Introspection and Awareness**

I concentrate on introspection to get insight into my beliefs, emotions, and behavioral patterns. Allowing me time to pause and reflect helps me identify triggers, case studies, and places for improvement. Using journaling, care exercises, or simply thoughtful contemplation, I cultivate mindfulness, which is the foundation of my mental well-being.

- **Deep Guidance**

## Falling In Love With Midlife

Midlife can evoke a wide range of emotions, including dread and vigor as well as sentimentality and vulnerability. I now know how to examine these emotions with empathy and recognition. Rather than suppressing or avoiding them, I allow myself to experience and express my emotions in constructive ways. This could be having a conversation with a trusted friend, practicing relaxing techniques, or engaging in creative expression.

- **Notable Connections**

Maintaining deep, meaningful relationships with those I love is essential to my mental well-being. I prioritize spending time with close friends and family, engaging in passionate conversations and intimate experiences. These connections provide me with a sense of belonging, support, and validation, which helps me remain resilient under trying circumstances.

Falling In Love With Midlife

- **Comprehensive Self-care**

Taking care of oneself includes all-encompassing activities that support my body, mind, and spirit; it goes beyond bubble baths and back rubs. I emphasize regular exercise, a healthy diet, enough sleep, and relaxing techniques like yoga or meditation. Engaging in activities that provide me joy and fulfillment, like gardening, drawing, or listening to music, revitalizes me and enhances my overall well-being.

- **Adaptability and Sturdiness**

Advances and changes characterize midlife, and I meet these head-on with adaptability and fortitude. Rather than resisting or fearing change, I welcome it as an opportunity for growth and restoration. This change in perspective allows me to maintain mental clarity even in the face of vulnerability, allowing me to explore life's highs and lows with beauty and idealism.

- **Seeking Guidance and Assistance**

I understand how important it is to ask for guidance and assistance when needed. Seeking assistance, whether from a trusted friend, family member, or mental health professional, is a sign of strength rather than weakness. Therapy, counseling, or teaching provide important tools and information to examine life's challenges and cultivate a more prominent mindfulness.

- **Boundaries and Self-Advocate**

Setting and adhering to boundaries is essential to maintaining my mental well-being and conserving my energy. In personal and professional relationships, I communicate my needs, preferences, and boundaries with decisiveness. This promotes healthy components and lessens stress and overwhelm, enabling me to maintain mental clarity and concentrate on the important things.

- **Engaging in Continuous Education**

My priorities are self-awareness and lifelong learning. I search for opportunities to broaden my perspective and point of view, whether it is by reading, visiting studios, or pursuing new hobbies. Learning stimulates my mind, sustains my curiosity, and builds my resilience in the face of adversity.

- **Respect and Attention**

Practicing gratitude and compassion is an essential component of my daily routine. I cultivate an attitude of gratitude by consistently acknowledging and appreciating the blessings in my life, no matter how small. Careful exercises, like mindful breathing or body checks, help me to center myself in the chaos of daily life and cultivate a sense of clarity and calm.

- **Accepting Yourself and Your Flaws**

I finally accept my flaw and engage in self-compassion. I recognize that I am fallible and that mistakes and accidents are inevitable. Rather than being judgmental or self-basic, I am thoughtful and compassionate toward myself, showing myself the same compassion I would extend to a friend going through a similar ordeal. This gentle approach promotes self-awareness and resiliency, which keeps my clarity and mental health intact as I navigate the fascinating turns and turns of midlife.

## What routines will help me maintain mental acuity?

Maintaining mental acuity in middle age is a complex task that calls for an all-encompassing strategy that takes into account various aspects of social, mental, and physical health. Keeping up with mental imperativeness is based on engaging in lifelong learning. This involves learning new material and efficiently testing your mental faculties with various activities. Gaining a new interest, learning a language, or delving into topics that pique your curiosity are all examples of how learning stimulates brain functions, increases mental flexibility, and fosters a development mindset.

It is equally vital to take action for mental health. Regular exercise improves physical and mental health as well as cardiovascular health and strength. Exercises that increase blood flow to the brain, such as cycling, swimming, or walking, help to create new neurons and improve mental function. Strength training and adaptation exercises also improve mental health overall by increasing brain resilience and versatility.

## Falling In Love With Midlife

Maintaining cerebral capacity and mental wellness needs sustenance. A diet rich in nutrients, minerals, omega-3 unsaturated fats, and cell reinforcements provides the brain with essential supplements that nourish the brain and prevent age-related mental decline. To fuel your body and mind, undervalue whole food sources such as veggies, whole grains, organic items, lean meats, and healthy fats.

Keeping your mind active also involves doing mentally stimulating workouts that test your cerebrum. Take part in activities that need critical thinking and deliberate reasoning, such as methodology games, puzzles, difficult but entertaining riddles, and exercises. These mental exercises help maintain cognitive function, enhance memory retention, and increase mental agility.

Maintaining strong relationships with associates is essential for overall prosperity, including mental wellness. Important social connections provide everyday comfort, intellectual stimulation, and possibly even doors open for academic dedication. Allocate a short period for routine social activities, such as spending time with family and friends, going on group outings, or attending community events.

Protecting mental capacity and promoting mental clarity can be aided by practicing care and stress management techniques. Mindfulness, deep breathing exercises, and yoga are among the care practices that reduce anxiety, enhance awareness and focus, and strengthen mental toughness. Incorporate these routines into your daily routine to cultivate a sense of calm and mental well-being.

Good sleep is essential for the health of the cerebrum and mental capacity. Don't repress anything that prevents your brain from getting enough uninterrupted sleep each night to allow it to rejuvenate and consolidate memories. Establish a comfortable sleeping environment and a calming sleep schedule to promote restful sleep and support optimal mental performance.

Lifelong learning and mental essentialness are promoted by keeping the mind engaged by reading comprehension, visiting addresses, and engaging in stimulating dialogues. To keep your mind focused and sharp, set aside some time for tasks that test your understanding and pique your curiosity.

Finally, seek out novel experiences to stimulate your mind and improve cognitive flexibility. Explore new hobbies, visit unfamiliar places, or take part in activities that aren't within your normal comfort zone. New experiences force the mind to adapt and grow, enhancing mental health and resilience.

## How can I create mental toughness and overall well-being?

This is an adventure that calls for thoughtful practices, mindfulness, and tolerance. Here are some specially designed solutions to help you become resilient and prosperous:

- Acknowledge Your Feelings:

Give yourself permission to express and feel a range of emotions, both positive and negative. Recognize that it's acceptable to experience weakness and ask for assistance when needed.

- Develop Self-Empathy:

Treat yourself kindly and understandingly, especially when things are tough. Treat yourself with the same compassion and understanding that you would extend to a loved one going through a difficult time.

- Discover Significance and Purpose:

Examine the things in your life that are important and purposeful. Engage in activities that are consistent with your traits and passions, such as lending a hand, looking for a creative pastime, or spending time in nature.

- Develop wholesome survival skills:

Recognize appropriate responses to particularly trying situations that help you manage stress and regulate your emotions. This could include caring exercises, real-world activities, writing, or seeking out qualified assistance.

- Establish Firm Relationships:

**Falling In Love With Midlife**

Maintain consistent relationships with friends, family, and neighbors that encourage and accept you. Making meaningful connections helps one feel supported and like one belongs when things are tough.

- Set Reasonable Goals:

Divide more ambitious goals into smaller, more manageable milestones and recognize your progress along the way. Establishing realistic expectations for yourself helps you avoid feeling in control and fosters a sense of accomplishment.

- Develop an Appreciation Practice:

Every day, take a moment to reflect on the things, no matter how small, you have to be grateful for. You can change your perspective and feel more prosperous by adopting an appreciative mindset.

- Embrace Change:

**Falling In Love With Midlife**

Recognize that change is an inevitable part of life and place an emphasis on changing with fortitude and flexibility. Seeing change as an opportunity for growth and education might help to lessen feelings of vulnerability.

- Set priorities Self-care:

Make self-care a priority by engaging in activities that support your body, mind, and spirit. This can include getting enough sleep, consuming wholesome foods, practicing relaxing techniques, and scheduling enjoyable exercise.

- Seek Help When Needed:

If you're struggling, don't hesitate to ask friends, family, or mental health professionals for assistance. Asking for assistance demonstrates strength, awareness, and togetherness.

# Chapter Eight

## Enhance My Cognitive Abilities

Improving cognitive abilities in middle age is essential for maintaining intelligence, adaptability, and overall profitability. Here is a detailed list of actions you can take at this ground-breaking stage to improve your cognitive abilities:

- Lifelong Learning:

Realizing the importance of continuous education, I actively sought out worthwhile opportunities to broaden my perspective and skill set. Whether it was attending local chat groups, attending studios, or enrolling in online classes, I welcomed lifelong learning as a way to challenge my brain and stimulate cognitive development.

- Practicing Mental Exercises:

**Falling In Love With Midlife**

I incorporated common mental exercises into my regular practice to maintain mental acuity. This involved solving puzzles, engaging in mind-numbing games, and doing activities that required critical thought and decisive reasoning. These psychological workouts helped me improve my memory and concentration, as well as stay up with cognitive dexterity.

- Eating a Solid Cerebrum Diet:

Recognizing the link between nutrition and mental capacity, I made informed choices to feed my brain foods high in supplements. I concentrated on developing a diet rich in whole grains, organic produce, lean meats, healthy fats, and little processed and sugary foods. Combining foods rich in minerals, omega-3 unsaturated fats, and cancer-prevention medicines maintained brain health and improved cognitive function.

- Regular Actual Exercise:

Realizing the many benefits of exercise, I concentrated on doing regular actual work to support mental health. Combining a variety of strenuous exercises, strength training, and flexibility techniques improved my physical health and increased blood flow to my brain, which improved cognitive function and brain adaptability.

- Prioritizing Quality Sleep:

I made rest a daily priority because I knew how important it was for cognitive function. Creating a relaxing sleep schedule and a consistent sleep schedule helped me achieve the recommended 7-9 hours of quality sleep every night for optimal mental health.

- Managing Stress:

**Falling In Love With Midlife**

Realizing the detrimental effects of persistent weight on mental capacity, I used pressure-free techniques to promote mental well-being. This included deep breathing exercises, relaxation techniques, and rehearsal care to reduce anxiety and enhance mental clarity.

- Remaining Socially Active:

Aware of the cognitive benefits of social collaboration, I made a concerted effort to maintain my social vitality and maintain my strengths with friends, family, and neighbors. Engaging in meaningful conversations, engaging in group activities, and seeking daily consolation from family and friends provided mental stimulation and a sense of community.

- Embracing Novel Experiences:

**Falling In Love With Midlife**

I looked for challenging situations and ingenious encounters to stimulate my brain and improve brain adaptability. Challenging assumptions, trying novel pastimes, or picking up new skills were all examples of how embracing curiosity opened doors to intellectual stimulation and cognitive growth.

- Continuously Testing Myself:

Realizing the importance of cognitive challenges in staying up with intelligence, I successfully looked for opportunities to push my mental limits. This involved tackling challenging duties at work, taking part in talks or chats about thought-provoking topics, and pursuing personal hobbies that called for creative thinking and decisive reasoning.

- Seeking Effective Guidance:

Realizing the value of professional assistance, I sought advice from subject matter specialists in cognitive science and emotional health when needed. Seeking expert guidance helped me be proactive in maintaining my cognitive well-being, whether it was to treat specific cognitive concerns or search for methods to enhance cognitive abilities.

I was able to maintain my intelligence in middle age and improve my cognitive abilities by incorporating these techniques into my daily routine. Adopting a holistic approach to managing brain health, I concentrated on lifelong learning, real work, stress management, social responsibility, and self-care to support cognitive function and overall success.

## How can I engage in mental health issues and lifetime learning?

Engaging in lifelong learning and mental challenges is not just a strategy to maintain mental acuity in midlife, but it's also a fulfilling endeavor that has the potential to significantly enhance your life. You can accept mental health issues and lifelong learning in this way:

*Embrace Interest:* Form an insatiable curiosity and an interested mindset. Approach life with an open mind and be willing to explore novel concepts, ideas, and experiences. The engine of lifelong learning and mental growth is interesting.

*Read Widely*: Develop the habit of regularly reading and exploring a variety of subjects, genres, and authors. Reading books of any kind, be it fiction, nonfiction, memoirs, or papers, broadens your vocabulary, sparks your imagination, and exposes you to different viewpoints.

*Attend Courses and Studios:* Enroll in workshops, studios, or courses that pique your interest. Many universities, community colleges, and online schools provide an extensive range of courses spanning from science and history to literature and art. Enrolling in classes enables you to develop new skills and broaden your understanding of specific areas.

***Attend discussions and Talks:*** Keep an eye out for public events and discussions taking place in your area. Speakers addressing current issues, new research findings, and social patterns are regularly featured in colleges, libraries, and social organizations. Attending addresses exposes you to novel ideas and sparks intellectual conversation.

***Participate in Conversation meetings***: Attend book clubs, conversation meetings, or online debates to engage in stimulating dialogue with like-minded others. Examining books, articles, or current events with like-minded others broadens your perspective and improves your ability to understand difficult concepts.

**Falling In Love With Midlife**

***Follow Your Imaginative and Side Interests:*** Look into creative pursuits and pastimes that will test your mental faculties and showcase your inventiveness. Painting, gardening, taking pictures, or practicing an instrument are examples of creative endeavors that stimulate the mind and provide a sense of fulfillment.

***Explore and Travel:*** Visiting new places exposes you to a variety of cultures, languages, and ways of life. Examine fresh objections, immerse oneself in local customs, and welcome fresh experiences. Traveling broadens your viewpoint and broadens your perspective.

***Remain Informed***: Accept innovation as a tool for research and education. Use online resources, educational software, and digital libraries to access a wealth of easily accessible information. Innovation creates many opportunities for lifelong learning, whether it's exploring virtual galleries, mastering a new language, or becoming an expert in something else.

***Push Yourself***: Look for academic challenges that force you to step beyond your comfort zone and foster personal growth. Solve riddles, solve puzzles, or learn a new skill that calls for mental effort. Accepting challenges stimulates the intellect and builds resilience and adaptability.

***Teach and Guide Others:*** Tutor or instruct others, sharing your knowledge and skills with them. Teaching benefits others and aids in your growth, whether you're teaching a younger partner, running a studio, or pitching in as a coach.

***Reflect and Survey:*** Set aside some time to consider your realizations and how they have enhanced your life. Keep a journal or blog to share your observations, insights, and experiences. You can maintain your caution and enthusiasm for the value of lifelong learning by taking into account your learning process.

## What activities promote mental agility and creativity?

It takes more than simply mental exercises to develop mental agility and creativity in middle age. You also need to engage in activities that spark interest, encourage self-expression, and ignite passion. Here's a closer look at certain workouts that can help improve these cognitive abilities at this revolutionary stage:

***Play Brain Preparation activities:*** Engage in brain-training activities such as logic puzzles, Sudoku, and crosswords. From my perspective, solving puzzles isn't the only thing I enjoy about it—I also enjoy the thrill of conquering challenges, honing my critical thinking skills, and experiencing a sense of accomplishment after solving a riddle.

***Picking Up an Instrument:*** Have you ever yearned to play the drums, guitar, or piano? The best time to pursue your dream is around midlife. Learning to play an instrument feeds your spirit and exercises your brain. I experience a deep sense of connection with the music when I pluck the strings of my guitar or hit the keys of a piano, and a wave of creativity flows through me.

***Artistic articulation:*** Using your creativity to its fullest potential through painting, drawing, chiseling, or creating is a powerful way to unleash your inner artist. I feel liberated when I pick up a paintbrush or mold soil with my hands because I'm translating my thoughts and emotions into a visual format and creating something truly unique.

**Falling In Love With Midlife**

*Writing*: I can release all of my stories, opinions, and feelings onto the paper when I write. It's my safe place. Writing helps me to explore the depths of my imagination, express my ideas authentically, and get perspective on my surroundings, whether I'm writing poetry, a short story, or a journal entry about my day.

*Dance or Development:* Development is a powerful form of self-articulation and creativity, whether it's practicing yoga in a serene studio or dancing to your favorite music in your family room. When I lose myself in the music of a dance or a yoga class, I experience a release of creative and motivational energy and a sense of liberation as my body moves in unison with my breath.

*Travel and Research:* Taking on new challenges makes me more aware of the world's wonders and piques my curiosity about them. Every new encounter I have broadens and expands my perspective and sparks novel ideas, whether I'm wandering around cobblestone streets in Europe, traveling through lush rainforests in South America, or contemplating ancient ruins in Asia.

***Dealing with Difficulties:*** Critical thinking exercises provide stimulating opportunities to examine my mental abilities, from escape rooms to riddles. I get a rush of adrenaline and a sense of camaraderie from working with others to solve puzzles and crack codes. We collaborate, strategize, and celebrate our collective successes.

***Reading and Acquiring Understanding:*** One of the simple pleasures of life is curling up with a good book. Whether I'm immersing myself in a thought-provoking real book, diving into a brilliant novel, or learning about the intricacies of physics and history, reading stimulates my creativity, broadens my perspective, and inspires me to think differently.

# Chapter Nine

## How Quickly will I Embrace Change and New Beginnings?

People often have established schedules, relationships, and personalities at this point in their lives, which makes the prospect of change daunting. Nevertheless, midlife may also be a time of great transformation and growth, with opportunities to welcome fresh experiences and redefine oneself.

**Comprehending the Midlife Transition**

Midlife, defined as the age range of 40 to 65, is largely defined by significant life events, such as changing careers, children leaving the nest, or improvements in health. These events can make one reevaluate the purpose and meaning of life. depicted midlife as a time of individuation, combining several aspects of oneself to achieve wholeness.

## Falling In Love With Midlife

Accepting change at this time means being open to new possibilities and willing to confront and let go of outdated aspects of one's identity.

## Elements Influencing the Massive Shift

Several factors can influence the speed and effectiveness of a person's midlife transformation:

1. *Mentality and Behavior*: Adapting to change can be made easier with a development mentality, which views obstacles as opportunities for growth and learning. Those who view midlife transitions as a chance for personal growth will undoubtedly adapt quickly and welcome new beginnings.

2. *Support Frameworks*: Having strong ties to family, friends, and partners can provide both practical and nearby assistance during times of transition. This support can strengthen confidence and adaptability, making it easier to investigate novel situations.

3. *Previous Experiences:* One's viewpoints and responses can be influenced by prior experiences with change. Those who have successfully navigated previous transitions may have greater confidence in their ability to handle upcoming ones. Conversely, unpleasant experiences might inspire fear and resistance.

4. *Health and Prosperity*: An individual's ability to adapt to change is significantly influenced by their level of physical and emotional well-being. It is easier to accept new beginnings when one is well, as they are frequently livelier and more optimistic. However, problems with well-being can increase stress and limit adaptability.

## Methods for Accepting Change

1. *Fostering a Positive Attitude*: It might help to shift focus from fear of the unknown to excitement for new opportunities by practicing kindness and

gratitude. Establishing realistic goals and acknowledging minor victories can also help to build momentum and confidence.

2. *Asking for Assistance:* Skilled advocates, life mentors, or assistance groups can provide guidance and encouragement. Giving experiences to people going through similar changes helps foster a sense of community and lessen feelings of isolation.

3. *Lifelong Learning*: Adopting a lifelong learning philosophy might help make adapting to change more reasonable. Thiscan entail picking up new hobbies, enrolling in educational programs, or searching for opportunities for professional growth. Continuous learning maintains the brain flexible and receptive to novel ideas.

4. *Self-Care*: Strength can be enhanced by concentrating on one's physical and domestic well-being through regular exercise, a healthy diet, and enough sleep. Meditation, yoga, and journaling

are among the techniques that might reduce stress and promote mental clarity.

5. ***Flexibility and Persistence***: Managing presumptions can be facilitated by realizing that change is a cycle rather than an isolated event. Relating to oneself with self-control and realizing that change involves some work can reduce discontent and anxiety.

**Change Has a Few Benefits:** It can spur progress. Even though the terms "change" and "development" are occasionally used synonymously, they are not the same. Change, in any case, can spur progress—a gradual ascent to a higher state—because it is a new beginning. It creates endurance since it involves letting go of the past and moving toward a new path. When change is difficult and you come out on the other side, you may look a little worse for wear, but you made it through, and that's what makes you a survivor. Enjoy your fortitude and tenacity; it disrupts the daily routine. Imagine spending your entire life doing the same thing in the same way at the same time: consuming the same meal, dressing similarly, and engaging in comparable activities. Please excuse me as I yawn. Tedium is so bland, so tasteless. If nothing changed, life would be a big sleeper.

It's an internal process of being that crosses the psyche, body, and soul and necessitates a transformation of the self. "Who am I as I exemplify this outer change?" it asks us.

**Three stages are typically distinguished in the transition interaction:** Consummation, Transitional stage, and, finally, fresh start. Below is a brief synopsis of each step, along with information on its attributes, methodology, and important questions to research at that phase.

**1  Finishing** - When something changes and something is lost as a result, this stage begins. We're being asked to give up our former selves, but we have no idea who we'll become yet.

- *Characteristics*: Pain, disorder, and discontent. This can be mixed in with happiness when the change is our choice or coincides with a happy event, such as a marriage, career promotion, or the arrival of a child.

- *Procedure*: Give yourself time to identify and process the emotions you experience when a situation ends; practice modifying your ways of letting go of things that no longer serve you while honoring what has gotten you this far; and accept that you may feel overwhelmed or in conflict when faced with a new situation.

- ***Questions to ponder:*** How can I honor the persona I'm portraying in addition to those or things who have supported me? Where am I holding onto things that are no longer useful, and how can I let them go? Where have I seen this before, and how can I use the lessons I've learned?

**2. Transition** - This phase can be described as a liminal state in which we have given up on the natural but are still unable to establish a new foundation.

- ***Features:*** Overpowering, Tension, Vulnerability. It may be assumed that even while we quickly adjust to our new roles—as a partner, boss, or parent, for example—our personalities, motivations, and working methods still lag. In the unlikely event that you are welcoming this change, it may also be a time of vigor, creativity, and growth.

- *Method*: Tolerance. While this is an important season for research, it can also be rushed with a sense of, "Are we there yet?!" Give yourself a chance to lay a solid foundation by concentrating more on long-term gains and less on short-term triumphs.

- *Questions to think about:* How can I give myself the time I truly desire to study and move through this phase at the appropriate pace? How could I let myself become unaware? How can I take care of myself to ensure that I have the endurance and flexibility that I truly desire?

**3. Beginning** - At this point, you have left the transitional area, fully accepted your new situation, and created new timetables and examples of living to support it.

- *Qualities*: Rejuvenation, vigor, power. You may feel as though you've fully embraced your new persona and have overcome your seasickness.

- *Method*: Take advantage of this time of life and new beginnings. Make every possible realization. Prepare for the next time the exchange will take place again.

- *Questions to think about*: What new legitimacy did this interaction give me? What skills and knowledge have I gained from this change? How could I prepare for the next time?

Transitions are an essential aspect of existence. We see them all the time in the natural world: the sun comes up and sets, the tides come in and go out, and the trees bud in the spring and shed their leaves in the pre-winter months. Generally speaking, normal change is progressive, occasionally surprising, and always unprotected from what already exists.

I was listening to someone talk about how they saw a group of geese take off while they were on a crowded cruise just yesterday. The birds took off in unison, and the tourists let forth a gasp of sheer amazement. In addition, the speaker posed the question, "Why does this experience affect our collective soul?"

He chose it because he believed it exploited our capacity for transformative reasonableness, which allows us to understand how birds could interpret the irregularities in life. September arrived in the north, and it was time for the gang to set out on its southern adventure. The birds were in the transitional state of moving to a new location in preparation for the upcoming season, as summer was coming to an end. This kind of frequent transparency can benefit us.

**Falling In Love With Midlife**

Change is unavoidable. It is up to you how you get from one stage of life to the next. Give yourself enough time, allow yourself to feel your emotions, double down on self-care, and seek assistance. In the unlikely event that you succeed, you'll feel strengthened and ready for a new beginning the next time you find yourself standing in the background of another city, getting ready for your big moment.

## What can I do to confidently navigate life transitions?

**From Misery To Fulfillment**

Moving from early adulthood to midlife is not as difficult as some people may think. For some, there is no hope for the transformation. They experience a lot of stuckness and slowness. With life, they grow apart. They no longer have a sense of identity, rationality, or connection to the larger community.

## Falling In Love With Midlife

To investigate midlife life transitions with confidence, a variety of approaches that prioritize organization, flexibility, mindfulness, and versatility are used. Large-scale changes are often brought about by midlife, including changes in one's career, family dynamics, health issues, and important opportunities to develop self-awareness. It takes thinking about, organizing, and supporting these changes.

First and foremost, it is critical to understand the concept of midlife transitions and believe that they are a normal aspect of life. Transitions that are common include changing careers, children moving out of the house, changing relationships through divorce or remarriage, and adjusting to parents who are becoming older. Normalizing these situations can help to reduce tension and feelings of imprisonment. When people realize that it's okay to feel suspicious or experience a crisis in their middle years, they can view these challenges as possible opportunities for personal growth.

During this time, mindfulness is essential. Taking a personal inventory helps you identify your strengths, weaknesses, achievements, and areas that still need work. Thinking about your work, relationships, health, and personal fulfillment can help you see where you are in life and where you need to go. Practices such as journaling, care, and reflection can help with transition-related emotions and increase mindfulness.

Midlife is a common time for career shifts, whether due to retirement planning, a desire for a change, or scaling down. It is essential to assess how well your current career is fulfilling and aligned with your goals and attributes. A smooth transition can be achieved by differentiating new skills needed for prospective career changes and allocating resources for training or preparation. Reconnecting with former partners and extending professional organizations might lead to new opportunities, therefore organizing is essential. Engaging with a career mentor can provide valuable guidance and support in developing a comprehensive transition strategy.

Prosperity and well-being start to matter more and more in midlife. Maintaining good health requires regular check-ups and screenings, a healthy diet, regular exercise, and enough sleep. It is important to seek treatment or advice for emotional well-being, and it is beneficial to practice pressure management techniques with executives. Having enough life, health, and disability protection provides inner peace and security.

Another fundamental aspect is the monetary arrangement. By completing a thorough assessment of your financial situation, which includes liabilities, retirement assets, and reserve funds, you understand your financial health. Creating or updating a budget that reflects your present and future needs, as well as improving savings and investment strategies with the help of a financial advisor, are wise decisions. Making sure you have adequate protection and inclusion is also crucial.

In midlife, family and marital dynamics may change. It is essential to communicate openly and honestly with family members about changes and their impact. Bonds are strengthened by spending quality time with loved ones and having a supportive network of friends and family close to home. Acknowledging the empty feeling that comes after the final child leaves the house and finding new activities or goals to focus on will help. If it's suitable, make use of this chance to get back in touch with your partner and look into common interests. Maintaining regular communication with children helps to sustain areas of strength for with.

Managing guardians who are maturing might be difficult. It is imperative that future needs, such as housing and healthcare, be planned for. Finding resources in your community or professional help to take care of you and make sure you take care of your health and prosperity is important.

Remarrying and getting divorced are significant life transitions that call for thoughtful planning and practical management. Getting help or attending support groups might help manage the close-to-home impact. Obtaining expert advice regarding legal and financial considerations ensures a more seamless transition. Focusing on creating a new life—dating, getting married again, or learning to love being single—can lead to fulfillment.

Changes in well-being could be expected as you become used to your new lifestyle. Changing one's lifestyle fundamentally, seeking out daily support from friends, family, or support groups, and closely collaborating with medical service providers to address any emerging or ongoing health issues are important phases.

**Falling In Love With Midlife**

Retirement planning involves defining your ideal retirement lifestyle, which may include activities, location, and manner of life. It is crucial to make sure you have a solid financial plan that includes investments, contingencies, and projected expenses. Being active and engaged after retirement is facilitated by planning for hobbies, volunteer work, or a side gig.

Strength from close to home is essential when examining midlife transitions. Building resilience strategies to deal with stress and personal upheavals, adopting an optimistic outlook, and relying on networks of emotionally stable people provide stability and strength. You remain curious and receptive to new experiences when you adapt and pick up new skills. Being flexible and prepared to change with the times helps one accept change as a necessary part of life and an opportunity for growth.

Extraterrestrial growth can provide direction and power. Internal harmony can be achieved by exploring otherworldliness or strict convictions, engaging with profound or strict networks, and incorporating care rehearsals into your daily routine.

Changing employment often means assessing responsibilities, assigning tasks when circumstances permit, and setting reasonable boundaries to maintain equilibrium and prevent burnout. Accepting innovation can benefit one's professional and personal life. It's helpful to stay up to date on new developments, make use of online resources and tools to learn new skills or manage daily tasks, and use technology to stay in touch with loved ones and professional associations.

Giving back in the form of mentoring, helping out, or setting up cultural events gives one a sense of purpose and fulfillment. Think about mentoring younger individuals, lending a hand to causes that are important to you, and reflecting on the legacy you must give up.

**Falling In Love With Midlife**

Adapting to tragedy involves allowing yourself to grieve and seek assistance, finding meaning and purpose in the wake of misfortune, and engaging in healing activities like therapy, support groups, or creative pursuits.

Regular introspection and reevaluation of your goals, progress, and life are essential. Be willing to adjust your goals based on the circumstances, and acknowledge and celebrate all of your successes, no matter how big or small.

## How can I open myself up to fresh encounters and adventures?

Midlife can be an exciting and remarkable time to invite new experiences and adventures. This time often offers a unique opportunity for self-discovery, growth, and re-establishment. Being open to new experiences requires a balance of bravery, purpose, and receptivity. Here's how you might approach this fascinating adventure:

First and foremost, cultivating an open mindset is essential. Recognize that midlife is a stage with possible results rather than a time of decline. Change your perspective to see this time as a chance to explore new hobbies, pursuits, and interests. To invite new experiences, you need to be open to change and willing to step outside of your comfort zone. With this perspective, you can be curious and ready to try new things without letting your fear of failing hold you back.

Next, examine your preferences and passions. Think of hobbies or pastimes you've wanted to pursue for a very long time but have put off due to other commitments. Midlife is the best time to revisit and indulge in these aspirations, whether they involve picking up a new language, purchasing an instrument, traveling abroad, or starting a new fitness regimen. Engage in activities that spark your passion and curiosity. This keeps your brain active and locked in while also advancing your life.

Developing a solid organizational structure can significantly increase your ability to welcome new experiences. Embrace a community of like-minded people who uplift and inspire you. Join networks, clubs, or get-togethers that share your interests. This opens doors for you and introduces you to new ideas and friendships. A vibrant network of emotional support can provide inspiration and solace, making it easier to embark on new experiences.

When dealing with new relationships, financial preparedness is assumed to be essential. Examine the situation to ensure that you may readily pursue new hobbies without undue strain. Making plans for travel, education, or new hobbies will help you make good financial decisions and experience new things. Speaking with a financial advisor can help with planning for these activities and provide a clear picture.

## Falling In Love With Midlife

Take care of your health and well-being to ensure that you have the vitality and energy to look into new projects. The essentials are regular exercise, a healthy diet, and enough sleep. A state of actual wellness can improve your ability to engage in various activities and experiences.

Mental well-being is also very important. Reflection, self-care, and yoga are among the practices that can help you stay grounded and focused, which will make it easier to greet new experiences with an optimistic outlook.

Accept the present and take on obstacles. Planning is important, but sometimes the most rewarding experiences come from allowing room for unrestricted endeavors. Always remember to say "yes" to any unexpected opportunities that present itself. Sometimes the most successful projects are spontaneous and spontaneous at the last minute.

Lastly, think back on your interactions. Write in a journal or blog about your new experiences, including the things you enjoyed and discovered. In addition to helping you value your experience, reflection can help you discover what truly brings you joy and satisfaction.

# VOCATIONAL LIFE

# Chapter Ten

## What Can I Do to Achieve Career Fulfillment and New Opportunities?

Midlife career fulfillment and new opportunities demand a comprehensive approach that includes introspection, upgrading one's skills, important planning, organization, and maintaining an optimistic mindset. You have the chance to align your work with your true passions and interests during this unique time. This is a comprehensive guide that will show you how to make the most out of this adventure:

**Deep Self-Examination:** Start by engaging in in-depth introspection. The middle years are a great time to reevaluate your professional path and make sure it aligns with your core values, passions, and long-term goals. Consider these methods:

- ***Identify Interests and Interests:*** Consider the activities and aspects of your work that you find most fulfilling. What makes you feel content and energized? Conversely, identify projects that help you focus your energies.

- ***Evaluate Your Achievements:*** Think back to your accomplishments and the aspects that you have found most enjoyable. This can help to highlight your strengths and areas of success.

- ***Assess Your Personality:*** Recognize what is important to you in your professional life. Is it flexibility, inventiveness, stability, making a difference, or something else entirely? Adapting your career to your strengths is essential for long-term satisfaction.

**Upgraded Skill Level:** Staying competitive and creating new opportunities in middle age requires updating or learning new skills. Here's how to proceed in that direction:

- ***Identify Expertise Holes:*** Consider your job goals while determining which skills you want to develop or advance. These could include industry-specific knowledge, sensitive skills, or specialized abilities.

- ***Invest resources in training:*** Enroll in degree programs, studios, affirmations, and online courses. Online learning platforms such as Coursera, Udemy, and LinkedIn Learning provide a variety of courses that can expand your skill set.

- ***Practical Learning:*** Take advantage of any opportunities for preparation that your manager may present to you. Offer your assistance on initiatives that will challenge you and provide learning opportunities.

- ***Training and Mentorship:*** Seek guidance from career mentors or tutors who may offer insights, feedback, and support in developing new skills.

**Planning:** Establishing and capitalizing on an organization's strengths is crucial to opening up new opportunities. The real approach to getting organized in middle age is like this:

- ***Reestablish Contact with Former Partners:*** Speak with former coworkers and superiors. Over lunch or espresso, catch up and review your career goals.
- ***Visit Industry Events:*** Participate in events, workshops, and classes. These events are ideal for networking with new people and staying up to date on industry trends.

- ***Join Associations with Proficiency:*** Join organizations with a clear industry focus and attend their events. This can grow your company and provide valuable resources.

- ***Make Use of Web-Based Entertainment:*** For system administrators, LinkedIn is a tremendous resource. Update your profile, participate in relevant events, and attract attention with posts and articles related to your industry.

**Guidance:** A mentor can provide valuable guidance and support while you investigate career advancements. The following is how to locate mentoring and benefit from it:

- ***Find Coaches:*** Identify those in your field who have successfully investigated similar modifications. Speak with them for advice and guidance.

- ***Formal Mentorship Projects:*** Appropriate mentorship programs are provided by several associations and expert affiliations. They can provide resources and structured assistance.

- ***Become a Guide:*** Sharing your knowledge and experience with others can be fulfilling and help you see things from other angles. Additionally, mentoring can strengthen your professional network.

**Examining Alternative Career Paths:** Midlife might often present an opportunity to explore whole new business ventures or career paths. Here's how to go about doing it:

- Run Informal Sessions: Talk to people in industries you're interested in. Learn about their experiences, the skills needed, and the challenges and rewards associated with their roles.

- Independent or Volunteer: Experiment by lending a hand or embarking on solo projects in a different industry. This can provide in-depth analysis and help you determine if it's a good fit.

- Research Projects: Devote time and effort to projects that excite you. Look for growth areas and think about how your skills might be applied to other positions.

**Budgeting:** It's essential to be financially stable when changing careers. This is how to plan your finances to create new opportunities:

- ***Examine Your Funds:*** Conduct a thorough assessment of your financial situation, taking into account all of your liabilities, responsibilities, and investments.

- ***Progress spending plan:*** Create a budget that accounts for anticipated shifts in expenses and income as your career develops. Consider keeping some extra money on hand to cover unexpected costs.

- ***Speak with a Financial Advisor:*** A financial advisor can help you prepare for the advancement of your career and ensure that you are making wise financial decisions.

**Maintaining a healthy balance between enjoyable and important activities:** A long-term career fulfilling balance between lighthearted and serious activities is essential. Here's how to make it happen:

- ***Mark your stopping points:*** Clearly describe your working and personal hours. Give your supervisor and your partners these boundaries.
- ***Concentrate on looking after oneself:*** Allocate a little time for activities that support your well-being—physical, mental,

and domestic. Regular activities, hobbies, and spending time with close relationships are important.

- ***Modular Work Paths of Action***: Look for flexible work schedules that allow you to truly balance work and personal commitments, if at all possible.

**Accepting Innovation:** Maintaining current with cutting-edge advancements might lead to new professional opportunities. Here's how to use innovation:

- ***Consistent Learning:*** Keep up with new gadgets and developments in your industry. To get better with technology, attend studios or take online courses.
- ***Computerized Presence:*** Establish and maintain key areas of a presence's power. An updated personal website and LinkedIn page

can showcase your skills and attract new opportunities.

- *Use Devices and Applications:* To streamline your work processes and expand your knowledge organization, make use of efficiency and systems administration applications.

**Accepting a Development Perspective:** It is imperative to adopt a development view to approach job transitions with adaptability and idealism. This is how to make it grow:

- *Accept Difficulties:* See obstacles as opportunities to grow and learn rather than as barriers. This perspective helps you stay resilient and strong.
- *Seek Input:* Request feedback from managers, coaches, and partners regularly. Make use of it to advance and grow.

- *Track Progress:* Acknowledge and celebrate your successes, no matter how small. This creates confidence and motivation.

**Defining Specific Goals:** Achieving career fulfillment requires setting realistic, unambiguous goals. This is how you should present and achieve your job goals:

- Clearly state what you need to achieve in your career when you describe your objectives. Clearly state your goals and make sure they are time-bound, appropriate, measurable, and attainable (shrewd).

- *Establish a Plan:* Develop a gradual plan to achieve your goals. Divide more ambitious goals into smaller, more manageable tasks.

- *Regularly Review and Adjust:* Review your progress from time to time and adjust your goals based on individual circumstances.

Keep your mind open to new opportunities and stay flexible.

## What professional goals should I set for myself?

Setting realistic objectives is a fun way to make sure you keep moving forward in your professional development and find fulfillment. Whether your goals are to advance in your current area, change occupations, or simply acquire new skills, setting attainable goals will help you stay on course. Here are some kind, tasteful suggestions for sensible midlife goal-setting:

It is important to consider the objective of aligning your career with your values and interests. The best time to think about what matters most to you is in your middle years. Think about the aspects of your work that you find most satisfying and the traits that motivate you. Perhaps you've always had a strong desire to assist others, or maybe you're drawn to creative pursuits. Adapting your profession to your principles and interests might lead to more inspiration and fulfillment.

Then, anticipate developing and rejuvenating your skills. The expert scene is always changing, so it's crucial to stay relevant. Determine which areas may benefit from more knowledge or skills. This could entail picking up new skills, enrolling in classes in emerging industries, or developing sensitive competencies like correspondence and administration. Investing in your education can keep you competitive in the job market and lead to new opportunities.

Establishing connections and managing systems should also be important objectives. Reputable professional associations can provide support, direction, and openings. Make it a point to get in touch with former business associates, attend industry events, and join associations for professionals. These connections may be important as you search for new opportunities or consider changing careers. Moreover, creating an organization may be enjoyable and enriching, giving you a sense of belonging and community.

Finding positions of influence may be a rewarding and challenging endeavor. In the unlikely event that you have accumulated a great deal of participation, think about how you might take on more responsibility and influence within your association or sector. This could include pursuing a promotion, spearheading an initiative, or mentoring younger colleagues. Important jobs enhance your CV and allow you to impart your knowledge and make a bigger impact.

**Falling In Love With Midlife**

Embracing flexibility and adaptation is another important objective. A key quality of every expert is the ability to pivot and adapt to changing circumstances. This could entail accepting autonomous responsibilities, researching remote employment opportunities that present incredible opportunities, or being accessible to growing organizations. Accepting flexibility might let you explore the changes and weaknesses that often come with midlife professional advancements.

Finding the right balance between enjoyable and important activities is crucial for long-term happiness and success. Midlife usually brings additional responsibilities, such as taking care of family members or managing health issues. Set goals that will allow you to genuinely make adjustments to your personal and professional lives. This can involve setting flexible work schedules, emphasizing self-care, or setting boundaries to ensure you have energy for relaxation and leisure.

Looking at different employment options may be a fun endeavor. Assuming that your current job isn't fulfilling you, think about what other businesses or careers would be interesting to you. To investigate different options, lead thought-provoking discussions, volunteer in new areas, or take up temporary work. Rekindling your enthusiasm and drive for work may occasionally be achieved through a horizontal shift or a whole professional makeover.

Security and financial readiness are essential objectives, especially when making plans for the future. Make sure your financial plans correspond with your work objectives and that you are on track with your retirement reserve funds. This can entail speaking with a financial advisor, altering the way you manage your investments, or setting up plans for future career shifts.

Continuous self-awareness should also be highly valued. Improvement of oneself is still intimately related to skillful growth. Set objectives to improve your capacity to deeply understand people, focus on executives and achieve universal prosperity. This could involve visiting studios, learning literature, or practicing mindfulness and caring. Enhancing your professional life via self-improvement might make you more resilient and adaptable.

In the end, consider the objective of providing something in return and making an impact. Midlife is a great time to consider what you can contribute to your community or industry. This might be offering guidance, lending a hand, or starting your initiative to address a cause that matters to you. Giving back can improve your professional process and provide a deep sense of inspiration and fulfillment.

## How can I explore exciting new career paths?

It's brave and exciting to explore new employment opportunities. This is your opportunity to reassess your professional approach, embrace your passions, and look for opportunities that align with your evolving values and aspirations. This is a comprehensive guide on the best way to investigate this revolutionary era:

**Consider Your Proclivities and Resources** Engaging in in-depth self-reflection is the most important step in exploring new job choices. This entails examining your tendencies, passions, and attributes. Consider this:

- What activities or pursuits make you feel content overall? Think about hobbies or interests you've needed to pursue professionally for a long time. Which facets of your previous or current roles have you participated in the most? Determine what aspects of your job provide you happiness and contentment.

- What core values do you uphold? Make sure that any new career aligns with these attributes, whether they are helping others, being inventive, or achieving financial soundness. Knowing your strengths and preferences allows you to make more informed decisions about future job routes that will affect you.

**Take Charge of an Ability Stock:** Make a thorough inventory of your skills and experiences. Enumerate the hard and soft skills you have developed throughout time, such as project management, administration, communication, and specialized abilities. Recognizing your strengths and flexible skills will help you see how they could be used in different projects or careers.

**Examine Potential Careers:** Once you have a clear understanding of your preferences and skills, look into possible job options. Make use of several resources:

- Industry Reports and Patterns: Look through industry reports to identify emerging industries with lots of opportunities.
- Work Sheets: Look through job advertisements to see what skills are needed and which positions are available in different locations.

**Conduct Educational Gatherings:** Meetings for education are invaluable for gaining experience in a variety of fields. Make contact with professionals in areas that interest you and request a meeting to learn about their experiences. Prepare questions that you can understand:

- What does an average workday look like for them?
- What challenges and honors do they have for their work?
- What skills and competencies are essential?
- What advice would they provide to someone considering a career in their field?

These conversations might help you determine whether a particular vocation is right for you by providing a realistic outlook on what lies ahead.

**Independent or Volunteer:** It is possible to gain in-depth knowledge in a different sector very quickly by outsourcing or chipping in. You can test things out without focusing on a full-time job thanks to these beneficial open doors. Look for volunteer opportunities or solo projects that put your skills to use in a different setting. This can help you gain a great deal of experience and make well-informed decisions about pursuing a certain course.

**Enroll in Classes to Earn Certifications:** Investing in further education can have a significant impact on switching careers. Acknowledge the essential skills and aptitudes needed for your dream career and pursue relevant training or certifications.

**Establish a Successful Network;** Establishing a robust expert network is essential while exploring alternative career pathways. Attend industry events, become a member of professional associations, and interact with online communities related to your area of interest. Systems administration can provide valuable connections, advice, and possible job prospects. Speaking with authorities in your desired field can also provide fresh perspectives and insights.

**Seek out mentorship:** Finding a coach with knowledge of the career you're considering might be quite beneficial. A tutor can provide guidance, support, and key information based on their personal experiences. They can help you explore the shift, avoid common pitfalls, and make important decisions.

**Examine several options regarding side projects.:** Starting a side project is usually a safe way to look into pursuing a different career path. If you're passionate about writing, for example, start a blog or submit articles to publications. If you're considering a profession in visual representation, build your portfolio by taking on freelance projects. With side projects, you can develop new skills, acquire knowledge, and amass confidence without having to quit your current job.

**Consider Your Financial Situation:** Switching careers might have financial consequences, so it's important to assess the situation and come up with a plan to handle the development calmly. This could be putting money away in a hidden stash, cutting expenses, or taking up part-time work while you make changes. Speaking with a financial advisor might help you create a financial plan that supports your professional objectives.

**Continue to be upbeat and liberal:** It can be challenging to look into new professional possibilities, but it's important to have an open-minded and optimistic mindset. Prepare for bad things to happen and see them as opportunities for learning. Stay flexible and willing to change as you learn more about the professions you're interested in and about yourself.

**Evaluate and Adjust:** Regularly evaluate your experiences and progress. Ask yourself:

- Are you enjoying the new activities and tasks you're engaging in?
- Do you feel your skills and strengths are being utilized?
- Are you excited about the prospects in the new field?

Based on your evaluations, adjust your approach as needed. This iterative process will help you refine your goals and move closer to a fulfilling new career.

**Take the Leap:** Once you have gathered enough information, gained relevant experience, and feel confident about your new career path, take the leap. This might involve applying for jobs, starting your own business, or enrolling in a full-time educational program. Trust in your preparation and take decisive action toward your new career.

# Chapter Eleven

## Balancing Life and Work?

Midlife career and life balance offer both opportunities and notable challenges. This time often comes with increased responsibilities, both practically and technically. Many end up at the top of their careers, firmly planted on senior footings that demand vital investment. Midlife can also mean increased family responsibilities, such as concentrating on helping parents mature, helping children through early education phases, or taking care of personal health concerns.

Setting up boundaries is a crucial step in achieving stability. In middle age, it becomes critical to separate work time from personal time to ensure that neither sector excessively interferes with the other. Setting up and adhering to rigid work hours can be beneficial. This can be turning off work messages after a certain hour or refraining from taking work home on Friday and Saturday. Establishing a dedicated workspace can also aid in maintaining this distance, even if one works from home.

Setting priorities is another fundamental component. Reevaluating needs is often necessary in midlife. Making the distinction between what is truly important in both personal and professional life can assist in center pursuits even more. This could be assigning tasks at work, learning how to say no to more responsibilities, or asking for assistance with personal issues. Spending less time on high-impact tasks and streamlining workouts can free up time for family, hobbies, and self-care.

In midlife, self-care becomes increasingly important. A healthy lifestyle starts with mental and physical well-being as well as deep reliability. Regular exercise, a balanced diet, enough sleep, and self-care exercises like introspection can all contribute to greater overall success. Additionally, midlife offers a wonderful chance to explore new hobbies or rekindle previous passions, which can provide a stress-relieving and revitalizing diversion from work

Maintaining open communication with family and friends is also essential. Discussing the need for offset with close ones can lead to more understanding and support at home. Having honest conversations about workload and efficient time management with coworkers or businesses helps foster a more stable work environment.

**Methods for balancing life and work:**

Achieving a harmonious balance between work and personal life in today's fast-paced and demanding environment is essential for both overall prosperity and career success. A key role in achieving some harmony is played by the board and

## Falling In Love With Midlife

viable career planning, which enable people to pursue their professional goals while maintaining a fulfilling personal life.This article explores the concept of work-life balance in career planning and provides helpful advice and methods for achieving congruence between professional goals and personal obligations.

### Recognizing Work-Life Balance

Work-life balance refers to a healthy balance between the amount of time spent on work and personal activities, such as family, hobbies, relaxation, and health. Achieving some form of balance ensures that people have sufficient resources for both professional and personal objectives.

### The Impact of Work-Life Balance on Vocational Planning

Professional planning is closely linked to work-life balance. An imbalance there can have a negative impact on one's career path and overall happiness. Through the incorporation of work-life balance into career planning, individuals can choose a path that aligns with their attributes and desires.

## Separating Needs from Objectives in Vocational Paths

Effective career planning starts with identifying specific career goals and requirements. Knowing what matters most enables people to make well-informed decisions and allocate their time and efforts accordingly.

Vati is a comprehensive career planning stage that helps individuals identify their needs and career goals. Vati assists clients in exploring their interests and tailoring their career options to their objectives through the use of its creative tools and resources. Using introspection and goal-setting, Vati helps individuals depart on a purposeful career path.

**Falling In Love With Midlife**

**Examining Personal Attributes and Preferences**

Personal traits and preferences are essential factors in career planning. Making career decisions based on personal traits enhances job satisfaction and fosters a sense of purpose in one's professional life.

**Understanding How Career Decisions Affect Work-Life Balance**

Some career choices may require more time and responsibilities, while others provide greater flexibility. Seeing how career selections affect work-life balance is essential to making well-informed choices.

**Set Boundaries and Concentrate on**

Setting boundaries between personal and professional life maintains a healthy balance. Concentrating on chores and exercise ensures that large investments are successfully appropriated.

**Employing Time Management Techniques**

**Falling In Love With Midlife**

The ability to manage one's time well is essential to achieving work-life balance. Techniques like concentrating on tasks, establishing reasonable deadlines, and getting rid of time-wasting activities boost productivity and relieve stress.

**Promoting Open Communication**

It's critical to communicate openly about the need for work-life balance with bosses and coworkers. Companies are beginning to recognize the value of employee prosperity and may provide flexibility or support.

**Accepting Flexibility and Working From Home**

In essence, flexibility and remote work options can improve work-life balance. Accepting these incredible opportunities enables people to schedule their employment so that they can more easily fulfill personal obligations.

**Falling In Love With Midlife**

**Innovation as a Tool for Proficiency**

Innovation provides a variety of tools to improve productivity and streamline workflows. Using correspondence stages and efficiency tools allows CEOs to operate effectively.

**How Important It Is to Rest and Look After Yourself**

Rest and self-care are important aspects of work-life balance. Maintaining energy and focus in professional and personal spheres requires taking breaks and making sure you get enough sleep.

**Maintaining Robust Relationships**

Good relationships with friends, lovers, and family contribute to work-life balance. Generally speaking, wealth increases when one surrounds themselves with a strong network.

**Developing Reasonable Presumptions**

Making reasonable assumptions about oneself and other people helps prevent feelings of overwhelm

**Falling In Love With Midlife**

and burnout. Maintaining a long-term career requires attempting balance rather than perfection.

**Highlighting Higher standards without sacrificing integrity**

Time well spent on projects, relationships, and personal activities is more significant than quantity. Prioritizing high-quality interactions increases customer and professional satisfaction.

**The Activity's Job and Real Health**

Having good health is essential to maintaining a work-life balance. In general, prosperity and energy levels are boosted by regular exercise, a healthy diet, and enough sleep.

**Attention and Anxiety The panel**

Practice care and stress management techniques are beneficial for reducing strain at work and improving overall flexibility.

**Falling In Love With Midlife**

**Expertise's Value Change in circumstances**

Investing in skillful progression increases career opportunities and opens doors while enabling people to balance work and life with increased effectiveness and knowledge.

Creating a Stable Work Environment Supervisors play a critical role in improving work-life balance. Higher work fulfillment and maintenance are encouraged by a stable work environment that emphasizes representative prosperity.

**Accepting Personal Interests and Leisure Activities**

Engaging in personal hobbies and interests outside of work provides a fulfilling outlet and contributes to a just way of living.

**The Benefits of Reaching a Work-Life Balance**

Achieving work-life balance has benefits that go beyond personal fulfillment. A balanced lifestyle has a significant impact on relationships, long-term career success, and overall health.

# How can I manage my time effectively to avoid burnout?

Managing time effectively to maintain balance in midlife is a difficult task that calls for careful planning and awareness. In many situations, midlife is characterized by a crossroads between enormous personal responsibilities and professional peak liabilities, thus adopting a complete approach to time management is essential.

1. ***Concentrate on Assignments***: The first step in using valuable time is to identify and concentrate on tasks. Sort assignments into four quadrants using techniques such as the Eisenhower Lattice: urgent and important, important but not dreadful, earnest but not major, and neither critical nor significant. Focus mostly on large-scale but insincere projects to prevent them from becoming crises.

2. ***Mark your stopping points***: It is essential to establish boundaries between your personal and professional life. Establish clear work schedules and adhere to them. During these hours, refrain from checking your messages or taking business calls. Protect your own time as well by scheduling regular breaks, outings, and alone time to recharge.

3. ***Assign and Cooperate***: Midlife responsibilities might become overwhelming. Determine how to assign tasks for doing errands at home and work. Put your family and group in charge of handling certain responsibilities. Working together reduces your workload and fosters a sense of accountability and support.

4. ***Exercise Taking care of yourself:*** Preventing burnout starts with taking care of oneself. Make sure your everyday routine includes enough sleep, a balanced diet, and regular

exercise. Engage in activities that promote relaxation and mental health, such as yoga, meditation, or enjoyable hobbies. Putting self-care first ensures that you have the stamina and adaptability to fulfill your responsibilities.

5. ***Time Impeding***: One effective way to increase productivity is through time impeding. Allocate specific time slots for different workouts throughout the day. As an illustration, allocate your mornings to high-demand tasks when your energy is at its peak, and your nights to social events or important assignments. Make sure to include blocks for solo workouts and relaxation

6. ***Learn to Say No:*** You may often receive numerous requests for a sizable investment in midlife. Understanding your boundaries and learning when to say no to additional tasks that could add to your workload are crucial.

Relatively turning down new projects or volunteer work maintains equilibrium and prevents overindulgence.

7. ***Apply Creativity Remarkably***: Use time management tools and programs to maximize efficiency. Task leaders, update frameworks, and schedule tools can help you stay organized and on schedule. However, be mindful of screen time and the possibility that technological advancements may interfere with personal time.

8. ***Ordinary Reflection and Change:*** Periodically consider the suitability of your time management procedures. Do you truly feel like you're in control? Is there a certain area where you constantly struggle? Modify your approach based on the circumstances, and maintain flexibility to respond to changing circumstances.

9. ***Seek Assistance***: Don't hesitate to ask a mentor, expert, or tutor for assistance. They can provide valuable insights and strategies for managing stress and maintaining equilibrium.

## What processes can help me achieve a fulfilling work-life balance?

Reaching a fulfilling work-life balance brings new opportunities as well as problems. This phase often involves examining high-level professional responsibilities while managing significant personal responsibilities, such as providing developmental assistance to growing parents and guardians. The following are step-by-step methods tailored for midlife:

1. Describe the needs and objectives Reevaluate Life Goals: Reevaluating your life goals is a great idea when you reach midlife. Consider what matters most

in your professional and personal circles, and adjust your requirements accordingly.

- ***Relocate to the center What Influences Change***: Concentrate on projects that correspond with your stated goals. Employ tools to identify and focus on important tasks rather than getting entangled in urgent but unimportant exercises.

2. Establish Strict Boundaries

- ***Work-Life Balance***: Clearly describe your working hours and free time. Avoid taking work home with you or sending depressing work-related alerts after hours.

- ***Dedicated Spaces:*** Establish a dedicated workstation if you work from home. The real division can aid in the cognitive differentiation of work and personal time.

3. Encouraging Time Management Time Hindering: Set aside certain periods for family, work, self-care, and recreation. Set out the mornings, for instance,

for high-boundary business errands, the evenings for get-togethers, and the nights for personal and family exercise.

- ***Apply Innovation Wisely***: Make use of productivity tools and software to manage tasks, create updates, and plan your schedule. Make sure screen time doesn't interfere with personal time by keeping an eye on it.

4. Assign and Reexamine

- ***At Work***: When possible, represent partners in endeavors. Assist your organization in taking on responsibilities to reduce your workload and foster a collaborative environment.

- ***At Home***: Reevaluate household chores like cleaning, mowing the lawn, or grocery shopping. This can relieve pressure and free up time for more intense workouts.

5. Pay attention to your own needs Actual Wellbeing:

Make sure you get enough sleep, maintain a regular exercise regimen, and eat a healthy diet. Real affluence is necessary to maintain focus and energy levels.

- Mental and Domestic Wellbeing: Engage in activities such as yoga, meditation, or leisure pursuits that promote relaxation and mental clarity.Make time every day to give yourself space to unwind and recharge.

6. Direct Communication

- *Family Conversations*: Be upfront with your family about the importance of maintaining a healthy balance in your life as well as your job obligations. Seek their assistance and support in managing your liabilities.

- *Workplace Transparency*: Communicate your boundaries and availability to coworkers and supervisors. Foster a culture that values personal time and encourages flexibility.

7. Learn how to refuse.

- ***Survey Responsibilities***: Consider how taking on more work or social obligations may affect your major investment before committing. Exercises that don't meet your needs or that can put you overburdened should be politely declined.

- ***Quality as the Center:*** Aim for greater standards in all aspects of work and personal dedication without compromising. Pay close attention to meaningful activities that make you feel good.

8. Typical Introspection and Modification

- ***Week-by-Week Scheduling:*** Set aside time each week to organize your schedule. Work, family, self-care, and leisure activities should all be included to ensure a well-rounded approach.

- ***Occasional Survey***: Consider your work-life balance regularly. Determine which areas need development and adjust your processes as needed. Because midlife is a special era in life, maintaining balance requires flexibility.

9. Seek Resources and Assistance

- ***Effective Guidance:*** Consider discussing midlife obstacles with a mentor, tutor, or expert. They can provide crucial information and strategies for managing pressure and achieving equilibrium.

- ***Influence Accessible Assets***: Make use of resources such as manager-provided health programs, flexible work schedules, and representative assistance programs.

10. Accept Flexibility and Flaws

- ***Adapt to Changes:*** Recognize that maintaining equilibrium necessitates ongoing engagement and flexibility. As circumstances and requirements change, be prepared to adapt your approach.

# Chapter Twelve

## How Can I Build a Lasting Legacy in My Professional Life?

Especially in your middle years, leaving a lasting professional legacy takes a thoughtful and comprehensive approach. You start by outlining your goal and motivation. Give careful thought to what you believe should be your professional legacy. Think about the influence you want to have on your field, your friends, and the larger community. It is essential to set long-term goals that support this vision. These goals should be clear, measurable, doable, relevant, and time-bound to ensure that they truly direct your actions.

Achievement in your field is another crucial component. Put your attention on long-term growth by staying up to date on the latest trends and advancements in your sector through conferences, certification programs, and courses. Strive for supremacy in your area of expertise by consistently creating and presenting original ideas that have the power to influence and change your sector.

Developing strong points is another aspect of creating a long-lasting legacy. Effectively mentor others by sharing your knowledge and expertise with junior staff members, assisting them in growing and succeeding in their careers. Organizing is equally important. Create and maintain a strong professional network by attending industry events, joining associations, and interacting with peers in person and virtually. Establish a cooperative work environment where people are motivated to collaborate, find each other's areas of strength, and build trusting relationships with one another.

It is essential to lead with validity and trustworthiness. Demonstrate moral leadership by making decisions based on reliability and sticking to your principles even in the face of challenges. Obtaining certification in your partnerships fosters loyalty and trust, two qualities that are essential for an enduring legacy.

Your inheritance gains an additional layer when you expand your local region. Engage in CSR initiatives that benefit the community, whether through giving back to the community, supporting industry-related social concerns, or engaging in philanthropic endeavors. Become known as the idea leader by imparting your knowledge through speaking engagements, writing articles, or book distribution.

Encouraging a strategy of advancement ensures that your legacy is coherent. Determine and support suitable heirs who can carry on your mission and core principles. Make sure all of your cycles, processes, and knowledge pieces are true to work efficiently and preserve your contributions for future use by others.

## Falling In Love With Midlife

Promoting a culture of positivity in the workplace is also important. Invest in representative improvement by providing training, opportunities for professional growth, and defined career development tracks. Promote a diverse and all-encompassing workplace, elevating other viewpoints and creating an atmosphere where everyone is valued and welcomed.

Progress and adaptability are essential to staying relevant. Keep your association on the cutting edge of industry innovations by embracing change and continuously seeking out ways to grow and advance. Encourage creativity within your team by fostering an environment where taking risks and experimenting with new ideas are encouraged.

Achieving long-term success and prosperity requires striking a balance between one's personal and professional lives. Execute manageable work practices that prevent burnout and promote long-term effectiveness and fulfillment. Make sureyour career goals complement your traits to enhance your overall sense of fulfillment and happiness.

To maintain and enhance your legacy, it's critical to engage in standard contemplation and advancement. Periodically assess your progress and influence, implementing basic adjustments to stay in alignment with your legacy goals. Seek advice from coworkers, tutors, and companions to hone and enhance your approach.

Finally, acknowledge successes and accomplishments along the way. Acknowledge your victories and those of your team, enhancing the beneficial influence you're creating. Tell people about your journey and your successes so others can follow your lead.

## <u>Which contributions might I possibly make that will have an impact down the road?</u>

Making a major difference in midlife involves using your resources, skills, and experience to create a lasting impression. Here are a few effective ways you can change things:

**Mentoring and Information Exchange**

Mentoring is one of the most remarkable methods to make a lasting impression. Reaching out to younger professionals with your knowledge, skills, and experiences can make a huge difference. You can influence the future of your sector informally by providing guidance and support to partners and up-and-coming pioneers, or formally through appropriate mentorship programs at your workplace or through associations for your industry. By investing in the betterment of others, you help ensure that your legacy endures via the advancement of the people you mentor.

## Falling In Love With Midlife

### Mental Prompt

Over time, you have accumulated a wealth of knowledge and experiences. By writing articles, books, or even online journals, and giving talks at conferences or seminars, you can establish a solid reputation for yourself as the subject matter expert in your industry. By exposing others to your innovative ideas and experiences, you can establish yourself as a formidable force that propels progress and inspires others. Long after you have left your professional position, your disseminated works might still inspire and educate others.

### Progress and Enhancement

In your sector, there has undoubtedly been a great deal of advancement. Focus on promoting progress inside your organization. Develop and implement new cycles, products, or services that have the potential to significantly improve client satisfaction, quality, or productivity. Leading the way in development strengthens your association's position and establishes new standards and rules for the industry, ensuring that your efforts are remembered and taken into consideration.

## Responsibility to the Community (CSR)

Engage in or initiate CSR activities that align with your abilities and proficiency. It can be incredibly satisfying to promote community networks, increase supportability, or advocate for social causes. You contribute to the prosperity of society and demonstrate your commitment to moral behavior by integrating your social responsibility into your professional work. These drives have the potential to positively impact networks and the climate.

## Creating a Culture of Positive Work Environment

Make the most of your background to create a welcoming and all-encompassing workplace culture. Promote diversity, value, and inclusion to ensure a stable, cooperative environment where all employees feel valued and included. A great workplace culture ensures that your influence continues to shape the hierarchical atmosphere, enhances representative fulfillment and upkeep, and sets the precedent for upcoming innovators.

**Important Charity**

Consider applying your resources, structure, and influence to support causes you care about via fundamental altruism. This can involve forming your establishment to address certain issues or acting on charitable boards or philanthropic alliances. You can make targeted contributions with vital magnanimity that have a long-lasting impact on society.

**Establishing Progression and Enhancing Authority**

Make rapid progress to ensure the coherence and manageability of your job. Determine and prepare future trailblazers who will be able to carry forth your mission and principles. Encouraging authority development opens doors and creates career paths that ensure your contributions continue to influence the industry and association even after you leave.

**Impact of Support and Strategy**

Make the most of your position and abilities to influence policies and advocate for reforms that will help your sector or society as a whole. Engage legislators, sign cautionary notes, and attend industry events to advocate for policies or campaigns that promote constructive change. Your assistance can lead to significant, dependable improvements in the way your industry operates and impacts the larger community.

**Environmental Custodianship**

Promote and carry out ethical behavior inside your organization. Promote policies and initiatives that reduce environmental effects, such as energy efficiency, waste reduction, and practical attainment. By emphasizing ecological stewardship, you escape from a heritage of maintainability and duty and contribute to the long-term health of the earth.

**Improvement of Oneself and Adaptability**

Finally, demonstrate your growth and adaptability. Describe the finest ways to balance personal riches with professional success, providing an example for others. By sharing your journey of overcoming obstacles and maintaining equilibrium, you will inspire others to pursue their goals with adaptability and a comprehensive approach to life.

## How can I share my knowledge and experiences with the next generation?

Contributing your expertise and life lessons to the forefront of midlife is a fulfilling way to support their growth and ensure the continuation of your legacy. Here are a few effective methods to achieve this:

Falling In Love With Midlife

**Projects for Mentoring:** Mentoring is one of the quickest and most efficient ways to share your knowledge. Look for appropriate mentorship programs in your industry or association. Offer to mentor younger colleagues or aspiring trailblazers, providing them with support, direction, and guidance. Your experiences can help them develop their skills, avoid typical entanglements, and explore their career paths.

**Teaching and Studios:** Consider doing a part-time stint at a local college or school. Many firms value the practical expertise and real-world experience that seasoned professionals bring to the homeroom. To offer your expertise on certain issues, you can also teach studios or classes through professional relationships or inside your association.

**Writing and Sending:** Write books, websites, or even articles to share your insights and experiences. Platforms such as LinkedIn, Medium, or industry-specific releases are excellent for reaching a large audience. Writing down your knowledge enables others to benefit from your expertise and has the power to inspire and educate readers long after it has been distributed.

**Speaking in Public:** Engage in open dialogue at events, seminars, and business meetings. Speaking to a larger audience allows you to share your experiences and knowledge. Speaking in front of an audience spreads your expertise and establishes you as a thought leader in your industry.

**Online classes and courses:** Create online courses or courses with themes related to your area of expertise. Anyone who is even somewhat interested in learning from you can access your information in an orderly and comprehensive manner thanks to online courses.

**Effective Systems Management Meetings:** Participate in or serve as the leader of expert systems administration associations and meetings. These conferences are fantastic for exchanging expertise, analyzing trends in the field, and mentoring upcoming professionals. Being gregarious at these kinds of events also helps you stay connected and continue to learn from others.

**Composing content for blogs and online entertainment:** Use your writing to give advice, experiences, and tidbits of knowledge on blogs and web entertainment. Regular posts on social media platforms can reach a large audience and spark dialogue. By Sharing your experience, lessons learned, and expert advice, you can inspire and educate future generations.

**Participating and nonprofits:** Donate your skills and time to charitable organizations that focus on education, youth development, or professional readiness. Many nonprofit organizations search for seasoned professionals to mentor children or provide training facilities. Your presence has the potential to significantly impact each member's professional and personal growth.

**Creating an Information Store:** Develop a knowledge base within your organization. This could be in the form of an internal blog, a series of educational videos, or a detailed manual. By reporting your cycles, systems, and experiences, you ensure that future representatives will be able to access and preserve your valuable expertise.

**Engaging in Organizations with Graduated Classes:** Participate in the graduated class organization of the institution where you received your diploma if you are affiliated with it. Many universities and colleges have initiatives that pair current students with graduates for career counseling and coaching. Your involvement can give students valuable guidance and opportunities for their future careers.

**Encouraging Informal Gatherings:** Organize get-togethers or lunch-and-learns within your association or neighborhood. These casual social gatherings can provide a forum for information exchange, industry analysis, and informal, friendly coaching.

# SPIRITUAL LIFE

# Chapter Thirteen

## How Can I Nurture My Spiritual Growth and Mindfulness?

A strong commitment to mindfulness, inner peace, and personal fulfillment is necessary to maintain spiritual development and awareness in middle age. Here are some specific tips and tricks to help you properly develop these viewpoints at this crucial stage of life:

**Introspection and Awareness**

- *Daily Reflection*: Make time each day for introspection, whether it is through journaling or thoughtful meditation. Examine your thoughts, deeds, and emotions to gain more insight into your behavior and sources of inspiration.

# Falling In Love With Midlife

- *Mindful Care*: Practice being present in the moment. Pay attention to your opinions and feelings without passing judgment. You can better grasp who you are and respond to situations with greater caution when you practice mindfulness.

## Meditation and introspection techniques

- *Normative Contemplation*: Make introspection a part of your routine. Start with brief meetings and increase the duration gradually as you gain comfort. To help calm your mind and improve your inner peace, focus on your breath, a mantra, or focused meditation.

- *Mindful Relaxation*: Throughout the day, engage in mindful breathing exercises. During stressful minutes, focus on yourself by taking deep, conscious breaths.

## Spiritual Reading and Research

- ***Dedicated Texts***: Peruse holy books or spiritual literature that aligns with your principles and beliefs. Think about the teachings and how you can use them in your life.

- ***Rousing Books***: Look for reading material that inspires and tests your spirituality. These can provide fresh insights and tidbits of information that broaden the scope of how you might understand your spiritual development.

## Taking Part in Nature

- ***Nature Strolls***: Make time each day to spend in nature. Walking in everyday environments can be a powerful way to connect with the environment and find a sense of balance and renewal.

- ***Careful Perception***: When you're in the outdoors, engage in mindfulness by paying attention to the small details, such as the sights, sounds, and smells. Through this program, you will become more grounded and develop a deeper connection to the everyday environment.

## Organizing a Daily Routine

- *Daily Ceremonies:* Establish routines that support your spiritual and mindfulness practices. This could include journaling about daily gratitude or engaging in morning or evening contemplation.

- *Consistency*: Ensure that your procedures are dependable. By being consistent, you may include these exercises into your daily routine and make them a defining aspect of your day.

## Creating a Stable People Organization

- *Spiritual Gatherings*: Become a part of a mindfulness or spiritual group. Attracting like-minded individuals can provide support, solace, and a sense of community.

- ***Studios and Retreats***: Attend studios and retreats focused on mindfulness and spiritual development. These intense experiences might enhance your education and impart fresh insights.

## Practice Expressing Thanks

- ***Appreciation Journaling***: Maintain a gratitude journal in which you regularly record the things for which you are thankful. This training helps you focus on the good things in life and promotes a sense of fulfillment.

- ***Expressing gratitude***: Develop the habit of expressing gratitude to others. Acknowledging and appreciating the kindness and assistance you receive strengthens your relationships and raises your sense of wealth.

**Falling In Love With Midlife**

**Engaging in Creative Activities**

• *Artisanship and Creativity*: Engage in creative activities such as writing, composing, or performing music. Expressing your spiritual experiences and interacting with your inner self can be accomplished through creative articulation.

• *Mindfulness through Careful Imagination:* Engage in attentive activities while using your imagination. Focus on the cycle rather than the outcome, allowing yourself to be fully present at that moment.

**Interrupting and Taking Over**

- Assisting others: Take part in acts of kindness or assist others. Helping those in need by canning provides a deep sense of inspiration and fulfillment and advances your spiritual development.

- Local Association: Engage in local activities that are consistent with your values and principles. Creating connections and enhancing the well-being of your community enhances your sense of belonging.

## Seeking Guidance

- ***Spiritual Tutors***: Seek guidance from mentors or instructors who possess spiritual insight and support for your journey. Their experiences and tidbits of wisdom can help you go on your exploration.

- ***Therapy and Guidance***: If you would like assistance in exploring other aspects of your spiritual development, consider therapy or guidance. A specialist can provide tools and perspectives to aid you on your journey.

## Adapting to Work and Personal Life

- ***Work-Life Integration:*** Attempt to strike a balance between your personal and professional lives. Make sure you dedicate a short period to mental and spiritual workouts.

- ***Mindfulness in the Workplace:*** Include mindfulness exercises into your regular workday. Take little breaks to practice deep breathing or introspection to help you stay present and focused.

## What spiritual disciplines can help me achieve inner peace?

Finding balance in midlife through spiritual activities can be incredibly fulfilling and remarkable. A few spiritual exercises that can help you achieve inner peace are as follows:

- **Considering**

Many spiritual activities are based on contemplation, which is particularly effective in promoting inner peace. Set aside some time each day to quietly sit and focus on your breath, a mantra, or focused introspection. This practice reduces stress, calms the mind, and cultivates a deep sense of inner peace. You may discover that contemplation leads to clarity and a strong sense of connection to your inner self as you get more comfortable with it.

- **Being mindful**

Being fully present in the moment and paying attention to your thoughts, feelings, and experiences without passing judgment are examples of mindfulness. Practicing mindfulness can be as simple as paying careful attention to routine activities like eating, walking, or doing dishes. You can develop a sense of harmony and contentment by focusing just on the present moment and reducing anxiety about the past and future.

- **Request**

Whether traditional or personal, supplication can be a powerful tool for connecting with a higher force or your inner wisdom. Praying normally to God can provide comfort, guidance, and a sense of connection to something greater than oneself. It might be a chance to express gratitude, seek assistance, and find solace in brief moments of vulnerability.

- **Yoga**

Yoga is a complete practice that promotes mental, physical, and spiritual well-being. It combines physical positions, breath control, and introspection. Regular yoga practice can help you develop your body's strong points as well as a calm, focused mind. Incorporating breath and growth can also help release tension and foster a sense of inner balance.

- **Writing in a Journal**

Writing down your thoughts, feelings, and experiences may be a wise and healing habit. You may manage your emotions, get insight into your behavior, and monitor your spiritual development by keeping a journal. It can also serve as a place to reflect on your spiritual journey, create goals, and express gratitude.

- **Practice of Appreciation**

**Falling In Love With Midlife**

Gaining appreciation can help you shift your focus from what is lacking in your life to what is abundant. Maintaining a gratitude journal, where you regularly record your blessings, can help you feel happier and more prosperous. This course can help you develop an inspiring outlook on life and help you value the moment that you are in.

- **The Nature Society**

Energy spent in nature has the unfathomable potential to establish and restore. Hiking, taking walks in the outdoors, or just lounging in a park can help you connect with the outside world and find a sense of balance and restoration. Taking in the beauty and patterns of the natural world can greatly calm you down and remind you of how intertwined everything is.

- **Spiritual Reading**

You can gain inspiration, guidance, and a deeper understanding of your spiritual path by immersing yourself in spiritual literature and writing that speaks to your convictions. Regular reading can uplift your soul and foster inner peace, whether it's sacred scriptures, poetry, or modern spiritual writings.

- **Administration and the local area**

Engaging with a community of like-minded individuals nearby can provide support, solace, and a sense of belonging. Participating in group activities, such as administrative projects, spiritual social meetings, or reflection sessions, can help you feel connected and contribute to a stronger sense of purpose. Serving others can also result in a deep sense of fulfillment and inner peace.

- **Services and Customs**

You can add meaning and design to your life by incorporating rituals and services. Be it lighting a candle, reciting a daily affirmation, or celebrating sporadic holidays, customs help you communicate your expectations, keep track of important moments, and connect with the sacred in your daily life.

- **Inhalation Techniques**

Practicing regulated breathing techniques, such as deep diaphragmatic breathing or alternate nostril breathing, can help calm the nervous system and lower blood pressure. Breathwork can be a very useful tool for developing a steady state of inner harmony and for receiving timely assistance when needed.

- **Skills in Handiwork and Creativity**

Engaging in creative endeavors such as writing, singing, or composition can serve as a means of expressing one's spirituality. With the help of these exercises, you can explore your inner world and communicate thoughts and emotions that might be difficult to articulate. Speaking creatively can be a thoughtful, restorative exercise that promotes inner peace.

## How can mindfulness improve my well-being?

Being fully present and participating in each moment without passing judgment is the practice of mindfulness, which has been shown to significantly enhance well-being, especially in middle age. During this time, experiencing many advancements and challenges—such as changing careers, navigating complex relationships, and developing self-awareness—is common. Regular practice of mindfulness can provide you with several benefits that enhance your overall well-being.

- **Reduction of Stress and Anxiety**

Stress in midlife can originate from a variety of places, such as obligations to family, financial concerns, and work-related responsibilities. By enabling you to focus on the present moment rather than worrying about the past or the future, mindfulness reduces stress and anxiety. Techniques like deliberate breathing and introspection, for instance, can trigger the body's relaxing response, lowering cortisol levels and promoting a sense of calm. You can cultivate a deeper level of adjustment and greater flexibility to stretch by practicing mindfulness regularly.

- **Enhancing the Nearby Guidelines**

As you navigate life's complexities, midlife can bring forth significant and significant changes. Being more aware of your emotions without reacting to them right away is one way that mindfulness enhances profound guidelines. This increased awareness enables you to pause and choose a more intelligent response to challenging situations. In the long run, mindfulness can lead to an improved ability to comprehend people more deeply, improved survival skills, and a more stable mindset.

- **Putting Real Health First**

Because of the robust mind-body connection, mindfulness has a discernible impact on your physical well-being. It has been demonstrated that standard mindfulness practice lowers heart rate, improves the quality of sleep, and lessens the aftereffects of chronic pain. Furthermore, mindfulness promotes a more apparent awareness of your body's needs, which helps you make healthier lifestyle choices. This increased awareness can lead to improved eating habits, more physical activity, and a reduction in harmful behaviors like smoking or binge drinking.

- **Encouraging Mental Capability**

Taking care of your mental health becomes more and more important as you get older. Studies have shown that practicing mindfulness can enhance a variety of cognitive functions, such as executive functioning, memory, and contemplation. You may educate your brain to stay on task and improve your ability to concentrate on projects by practicing mindfulness.Improved self-direction, critical thinking skills, and general mental imperativeness can all be prompted by this mental clarity.

- **Promoting Improved Interactions**

Relationships have a crucial role in well-being, and practicing mindfulness can enhance the quality of your interactions with other people. Practice thoughtful writing because it helps you be more aware and present in conversations, which promotes more connections and comprehension. By practicing mindfulness, you may lessen arguments and misperceptions while listening and responding with empathy. These enhancements can strengthen your relationships with friends, family, and partners, contributing to a stronger sense of belonging and social support.

- **Gaining More Self-Empathy**

Midlife can be a time of introspection and assessment of oneself, which occasionally leads to self-criticism and self-deprecating thoughts. Being mindful teaches you to be kind and patient with yourself, especially when things are hard. This cultivates self-sympathy. This compassionate perspective can lessen feelings of guilt and inadequacy, promoting a better mental image of oneself and more prominent self-acknowledgment.

**Falling In Love With Midlife**

- **Increasing Contentment and Fulfillment in Life**

Being mindful helps you appreciate the small pleasures in life and live in the moment. Focusing on the here and now helps you cultivate a sense of gratitude and contentment that underpins overall joy and fulfillment in life. Additionally, mindfulness helps you align your actions with your values and goals by energizing a sense of purpose and direction. This arrangement can lead to a very purposeful and fulfilling life.

- **Managing Midlife Transitions**

Significant advancements, such as professional shifts, unusual relationship dynamics, or individual personality traits, are often experienced in midlife. The tools to investigate these developments with ease and grace are provided by mindfulness. With an open and adaptable mindset, you can embrace change by staying in the moment and accepting each moment as it comes. This flexibility can help you meet challenges head-on and embrace new opportunities.

- **Enhancing Self-Reflection and Awareness**

Being mindful helps you understand yourself and your inner world on a deeper level. You can gain insight into your thoughts, emotions, and behaviors via regular practice, which will lead to more notable awareness. Being mindful can promote self-awareness and personal development, enabling you to make thoughtful decisions that are consistent with who you are. This might be particularly important in midlife when you try to reassess your needs and personality.

- **Advancing the development of work-life balance**

It might be difficult to adjust to professional and personal life, especially in middle age. Being mindful helps you set boundaries and keep your attention on your health. Being more aware of how you spend your substantial investment will enable you to make deliberate choices that will ensure a better work-life balance. Additionally, mindfulness increases effectiveness and efficiency, enabling you to fulfill your responsibilities with greater sincerity and carve out time for relaxation and leisure.

- **Encouraging Mental Wellness**

It has been demonstrated that mindfulness reduces the negative impacts of anxiety, depression, and other mental health conditions. Mindfulness helps you break free from negative thought patterns and reduce rumination by fostering a nonjudgmental awareness of your opinions and feelings. Improved mental health and a more notable sense of close-to-home well-being can result from this exercise.

# Chapter Fourteen

## Finding Purpose and Meaning

Finding meaning and purpose in midlife usually involves a deeper introspective journey because this is the time when many people reflect on their achievements, aspirations, and lifestyles. This is an itemized reference:

1. ***Consider Past Encounters***: Examine your past experiences, both favorable and unfavorable. Acknowledge moments of joy, success, and contentment in addition to challenges and errors. Think about how these experiences have shaped your wants, values, and beliefs.

2. ***Identify Basic Beliefs***: Describe your core values and principles, which operate as a guide for your decisions and actions. Think about what matters most to you in life: your

family, your work, your creativity, your
otherworldliness, your neighborhood, or your
self-awareness.

3. ***Investigate Interests and Interests***: Look into
fresh or old interests and interests. Think of
activities that pique your attention, make you
happy, and make you feel good. Look for
activities that resonate with your spirit,
whether they are in the form of writing,
music, art, athletics, or the outdoors.

4. ***Establish Meaningful Goals:*** Define
objectives that are consistent with your
interests and values. These objectives may be
professional, personal, or both. Divide them
up into smaller, more manageable tasks and
come up with a plan to do them.

5. ***Seek Self-Improvement:*** Seize opportunities
for personal development and self-awareness.
This could entail learning new skills,
pursuing further education or certifications,

or engaging in counseling or treatment to deal with personal issues and cultivate awareness.

6. ***Nurture Connections***: Form deep bonds with your loved ones, friends, and neighborhood. Invest in relationships that bring you joy, comfort, and a sense of belonging. Be in the company of positive and inspiring individuals.

7. ***Give Back Through Help:*** Look for opportunities to show others how much you care by lending a hand or being kind. Contributing to causes that align with your beliefs can provide a strong sense of fulfillment and purpose.

8. ***Accept Change and Versatility***: As you explore your midlife endeavor, be open to change and flexible. Recognize that meaning and purpose can evolve and welcome new opportunities for growth and exploration.

9. ***Show kindness and gratitude:*** Cultivate gratitude and concern in your daily life. Take advantage of the chance to appreciate the gifts in your life and the moment you are in. Practice showing gratitude can promote a deeper sense of contentment and joy.

10. ***Celebrate Your Excursion***: Take pride in your achievements, no matter how small, and acknowledge the progress you've made in your quest to discover meaning and purpose in midlife. Remember that the journey itself is important, and every move in the right direction is an expression of your adaptability and might.

## How can I connect with my deeper values and beliefs?

Exploring your deeper values and beliefs in midlife involves a multi-layered inquiry that calls for a balance of action, introspection, and contemplation. How about we delve more into each of the described procedures:

- Consider Your Life Path:

Look for opportunities to revisit significant moments in your life, both happy and unhappy. Think about how these experiences have influenced your decisions, molded your personality, and shaped your point of view. Think about the values that emerged from these experiences and how they continue to shape your wants and viewsto this day.

- Elucidate Your Core Principles:

Engage in a reflective process to identify the principles that resonate most deeply with you. Consider using exercises or prompts to explore your values, such as creating a list of your beliefs or visualizing your ideal memorial. Think about the ways these values show themselves in your relationships, work, health, and self-awareness, among other areas of your life.

- Discover Meaningful Moments:

Dive deeply into memories and experiences that have an enduring impact on your complete self. These minutes may include moments of devotion, connection, creativity, adaptability, or ethereal stimulation. Consider the fundamental topics and ideals that these interactions exemplify, and reflect on how you may use more of these moments to advance in your life.

- Practice Self-Disclosure:

Experiment with various self-revelation techniques to expand your understanding of your inner self and surroundings. Journaling, self-reflection, contemplation, and caregiving can all be highly beneficial tools for cultivating insight and awareness. Set aside regular time to explore your thoughts, emotions, and beliefs with curiosity and compassion using these activities.

- Evaluate Your Continuing Concerns:

**Falling In Love With Midlife**

Make a thorough evaluation of your continuing requirements and obligations to determine whether they are consistent with your guiding principles and beliefs. Could it be argued that you are investing in activities that bring you happiness and fulfillment, or would you argue that you are keeping up with obligations and diversions that take you away from what matters most to you? Determine the areas where you may need to realign your needs for them to be more closely in line with your values and objectives.

- Look to Job Models for Motivation:

Pay attention to those who inspire you with their sincerity, relevance, and commitment to their principles. These excellent examples could be well-known individuals, figures that can be independently verified, instructors, or specific coworkers whose lives reflect the values and traits you value most. Focus on their stories, insights, and logic to find inspiration and guidance in living a life consistent with your deepest principles.

• Establish a Spiritual and Natural Connection: Create a deeper connection with the natural world and the otherworld as a source of inspiration and replenishment. Spend time outside immersing yourself in the beauty and wonder of the everyday environment. Engage in spiritual activities such as introspection, prayer, or rituals that align with your beliefs and help you connect with a sense of grandeur, meaning, and unity.

• Embrace Development and Transformation: As you rediscover your deeper values and beliefs, embrace the path of development and change. Recognize that this journey may involve facing discomfort, vulnerability, and resistance whileyou look into new options and let go of outdated models or ideas that will never benefit you again. Accept challenges as opportunities for growth and learning, and have faith in your ability to overcome them and succeed.

- Seek Support and Accountability:

Surround yourself with a consistent group of friends, family, or guides who understand and value your adventure. Talk about your goals, struggles, and experiences with trusted individuals who can provide guidance, accountability, and support. Join forces with others who have similar ideals and aspirations to further your efforts and foster a sense of solidarity and strength.

- Apply Patience and Self-Empathy:

As you explore the nuances of getting in touch with your deeper values and beliefs, treat yourself with kindness and gentleness. Recognize that this is not a linear journey and that there may be moments of uncertainty, chaos, and challenges along the way. Develop self-compassion by acknowledging your efforts and advancements, and cultivate perseverance by allowing the process of self-discovery and transformation to unfold willingly.

You can go on a major journey of self-discovery and reconnection with your deeper values and beliefs in midlife by connecting really in these disciplines. Accept the cycle with openness, curiosity, and an openness to learning, understanding that it may improve every aspect of your life and result in greater meaningful fulfillment, sincerity, and meaning.

## What activities can help me feel more spiritually fulfilled?

Finding spiritual fulfillment in life's complexities becomes a uniquely stitched artwork of one's unique experiences, insights, and connections, especially when one investigates the remarkable scene of midlife. From my perspective, it goes beyond simply finding minutes; it involves creating a mindful environment in which my soul may resonate with logic and connection, transcending the mundane and connecting with the essence of existence itself.

In the middle of the chaos of daily life, contemplation has become my refuge, my safe place. Those quiet moments, when I find a distant corner, close my eyes, and surrender to the rhythm of my breathing, are when I have a deep sense of clarity and harmony within. Perhaps I'm peeling back the layers of disruption and chaos to reveal my deepest insights, which are at the core of who I am. Every breath I take and every breath out becomes a gentle reminder to release the worries and tensions that weigh me down and allow me to re-establish my connection to the essence of who I am and what matters most in life.

Nature, in all her infinite brilliance and cunning, will always be my greatest teacher and source of inspiration. Being immersed in the ordinary environment makes me feel amazed and loved, whether it's a solitary ascent through the surpassing trees of a dense forest or a serene stroll along the shores of an abandoned ocean side. I feel most alive and connected to the planet during those little moments of peaceful communion with it; it's as if every leaf, every patch of grass, and every wave in the lake are directly whispering intimate details of the cosmos to my soul.

I take solace in the embrace of an option that might be more important than me in these moments of contemplation and prayer. I have a strong sense of connection to the celestial, whether I'm sitting in silence with the sun filling my face or bowing in prayer with words coming directly from my heart. Perhaps I am exploiting a source of wisdom and love that reaches beyond the boundaries of this world to tell me that I am never truly alone on this journey through life.

All of the imagination's teeming structures have become my spirit's look, my way of imbuing significance and grandeur into the texture of everyday existence. Imaginative expression is where I feel most alive and connected to my true self, whether I'm writing a poem that flows across the page, painting with colors that sing, or hurriedly dancing beneath the stars. I feel the boundaries between the cosmos and myself dissolve at those moments of unrestrained self-expression as if I'm drawing from an endless supply of inspiration and credibility.

Kind deeds and compassion are the threads that bind us together as a society, tying together an affection and interdependence that transcends personal differences and divisions. These small acts of kindness, like volunteering at a local sanctuary, giving a neighbor in need a helping hand, or simply grinning at a stranger in the city, remind me of the power of love to heal and transform—both ourselves and our environment as a whole.

## Falling In Love With Midlife

In the peaceful moments preceding sleep, while I lie beneath the subtle glow of the evening, I also reflect on the blessings, big and small, that I have received throughout my life. I feel incredibly happy when I am shown gratitude for anything, from the simple pleasures of a warm cup of tea to the love I have for those I love, and it reminds me of the abundance that surrounds me every day. Those few moments of quiet contemplation are when I usually feel most closely connected to the essence of life as if each breath were a sacred prayer of thanksgiving for the miracle of existence.

Through these practices—and that's just the tip of the iceberg—I continue to journey toward spiritual fulfillment, understanding that while the path may seem pointless, the destination is always within reach, waiting to welcome me with open arms.

# Chapter Fifteen

## How Can I Give Back and Get Involved in the Community?

In addition to being particularly fulfilling, giving back to the community in midlife advances societal advancement and general prosperity. By the time we reach this stage of life, we often have acquired shrewdness, skills, and resources that can be valuable assets for our networks. In exchange, please consider the following.

- **Volunteer Open Doors:**

Look into valuable open doors that align with your hobbies, skills, and inclinations among neighboring workers. There are countless ways to have a positive impact in your community, whether it's volunteering at a local animal shelter, coaching young people, organizing environmental cleanups, or serving dinners at a soup kitchen. To find out about volunteer opportunities that fit your preferences and availability, think about getting in touch with community centers, charity associations, or strict establishments.

- **Join Community Associations**:

Get involved in organizations and campaigns within your community that aim to solve specific needs or problems. This might be becoming a member of a neighborhood promotion group, joining a local association, or joining a service club. You may increase your influence and make a big difference in your community by surrounding yourself with like-minded individuals and combining your resources.

- **Express Your Skills and Talents**:

Use your expertise and knowledge to benefit your community. Offer to conduct a workshop or host an educational session on your topic of expertise, be it innovation, healthcare, or something else entirely.

# Falling In Love With Midlife

Think about offering your time as a volunteer educator or consultant to individuals or businesses that want to grow and be successful. By lending your knowledge and experience, you can inspire others to achieve their goals and strengthen the social and economic fabric of your neighborhood.

- **Support Local Organizations and efforts**:

Participate in local markets and festivities, purchase locally, and attend community events to show your support for local organizations and efforts. By disparaging local businesses and investing in the local economy, you help establish your position, boost economic growth, and foster a sense of adaptability and community pride. Look for opportunities to collaborate with local associations and business owners to promote financial progress and development in your area.

- **Advocate for Social Change**:

Support initiatives aimed at resolving social problems and promoting constructive change within your community. Maintaining fair housing, racial fairness, environmental sustainability, or access to healthcare are just a few of the causes that can be supported, brought to light, and used to influence decisions made on policy at the federal, state, and local levels. Consider participating in or supporting grassroots initiatives, attending neighborhood or local events, contacting appropriate authorities to voice your concerns, and finding allies for arrangements.

- **Plan Community Events**:

Take the initiative and plan events and activities that bring people together and foster a sense of belonging and community. Organizing events can strengthen social bonds, build community strength, and promote city dedication, whether it's a neighborhood barbecue, a social celebration, or a community clean-up day. Collaborate with volunteer groups, neighborhood associations, and organizations to plan and carry out successful events that benefit the entire community.

- **Serve on Sheets and Councils**: Consider volunteering for local non-profit groups, governmental bodies, or community drives by serving on sheets, boards of trustees, or warning boards. You may help shape strategies, initiatives, and campaigns that tackle fundamental problems and improve residents' quality of life by contributing your time, skills, and managerial abilities. Look for opportunities to share your unique perspective and make a big difference in areas including education, healthcare, housing, and social services.

- **Take Part in Intergenerational Activities**: Through intergenerational activities and initiatives, build relationships with people of all ages and backgrounds. Volunteer to mentor, counsel, or simply be a friend to individuals of all ages at schools, youth organizations, or elder centers. Through bridging the generational divide and fostering meaningful relationships across different age groups, you can promote grasping, empathy, and social attachment within your community.

- **Promote Community Health and Wellbeing**:

Take part in campaigns that promote community health and well-being, such as organizing fitness centers, food studios, or support groups for mental health. Promote access to athletic offices, wholesome food options, and healthcare administrations in underprivileged areas of your community. By concentrating on your health and well-being, you may help improve your overall sense of fulfillment in life and the significance of your community.

- **Take the lead As a visual cue:**

Set a good example for community inclusion and civic commitment by demonstrating how it's done. Demonstrate your responsibility to make a difference in your community by your actions, words, and words. Encourage people to give back by sharing your own experiences, successes, and sources of inspiration. You may encourage a culture of management, liberality, and empathy that will sustain your community's social fabric for a very long time by demonstrating to others how it's done.

## What are the joys of volunteering and making a positive impact?

The experience of volunteering and producing a positive result takes on a deeply personal significance in midlife, wrapping around strands of development, affiliation, and direction that resonate with the embodiment of who I am and what I strive to be.

The sense of purpose and direction volunteering gives me is one of the greatest joys I've discovered in life. As I transitioned from the demands of a busy job to a more reflective phase, I found myself yearning for worthwhile opportunities to give back and make a real, meaningful impact. Serving meals at a neighborhood restaurant, mentoring a child who struggles with reading, or spending time with abandoned animals at a rescue center are just a few examples of how helping others makes me feel incredibly happy and fulfilled. It also shows me that the lives of those around me can be significantly impacted by the things I do.

Additionally, volunteering has given me access to a broad web of connections and a sense of community that have greatly improved my life. The sense of brotherhood and place I've found through volunteering has extended my feeling of association with my general surroundings and helped me to remember the force of solidarity in making good change, whether it's holding with individual workers over shared encounters, forging significant relationships with those I serve, or working with community partners to address pressing needs.

## Falling In Love With Midlife

I've also seen enormous personal growth and development as a result of volunteering; I've been forced to venture outside of my comfort zone, learn new skills, and broaden my perspectives in ways I never would have imagined. Whether it was overcoming my fear of public speaking by operating recording studios for young people in danger, learning how to investigate social differences and language barriers while doing volunteer work overseas, or discovering hidden talents and passions I never knew I had, every experience has helped me become a more understanding, resilient, and caring person.

I think volunteering has given me a renewed sense of gratitude and perspective in particular, which has inspired me to live a more generous, purposeful, and compassionate life by reminding me of all the benefits I have received. As I observe the struggles and obstacles faced by others in my community, I'm depressed by the abundance of resources, incredible opportunities, and networks of emotional support that I often undervalue. This increased awareness of my honor and favors has strengthened my duty to give back and serve others, which fuels my desire to see positive changes in my immediate environment.

Ultimately, the joys of volunteering and experiencing a positive outcome in midlife are deeply personal and immensely satisfying, reminding me of the magnificence and interdependence of the human condition and inspiring me to continue striving for a brighter, more compassionate future for everybody.

## How can I build a legacy through community service?

As I enter my middle years, I find that I'm more drawn to creating a legacy that extends beyond my achievements and has a lasting impact on my surroundings. From my perspective, community administration has emerged as a potent means of creating a lasting impact that aligns with my traits, passions, and objectives.

One of the most important ways I've discovered to leave a legacy in community administration is through wise financial management of my time, money, and resources, which I invest in causes close to my heart. Whether it's volunteering at a local food bank, organizing pledge drives for charitable organizations, or advocating for civil rights and environmental sustainability, every act of leadership becomes a thread in the tapestry of my history, wrapping around a tale of empathy, compassion, and duty to have a positive impact on the world.

Engaging in community administration means that I'm prepared to apply my knowledge, experience, and skills to meet pressing needs and contribute to the well-being of others. Whether it's using my professional foundation tutoring skills to help businesspeople, exhibiting studios on financial literacy and career advancement, or sharing my passion for craftsmanship and creativity with marginalized youth, every opportunity I get to make a lasting impression on the lives I touch, inspiring them to reach their full potential and realize their dreams.

Additionally, community administration provides me with a platform to foster relationships and build ties that transcend personal interactions and endure long after I'm gone. Whether it's creating bonds with specific employees, forming bonds with neighborhood associations and organizations, or mentoring the next generation of pioneers, each relationship becomes a cornerstone of my history, strengthening the social fabric of my neighborhood and inspiring others to continue the work that has been shaped by generosity and leadership.

I'm prepared to use community administration to foster a sense of ownership and belonging in the networks I support, fostering a spirit of collaboration, adaptability, and fortification that extends well beyond my pursuits. Organizing neighborhood clean-up events, renovating public areas, or advocating for policies that promote worth and thoughtfulness—all of these initiatives serve as examples of the power of group effort and the enduring legacy of community management.

Perhaps more than anything else, community administration allows me to model and impart traits that are typically important to me, such as empathy, morality, and a sense of duty to others. Every action I do, whether it's showing my children that I'm liberal and considerate, inspiring my friends to volunteer, or leaving an estate to support organizations that are important to me, leaves a lasting influence and serves as a beacon of hope for others.

# Conclusion

In "How to Love Midlife: Unlocking 15 Reasons to Loving Life in Your Golden Years," takes us on a profound voyage of self-discovery, growth, and celebration of the opulence that comes with reaching midlife. Through our examination of fifteen compelling reasons to welcome this revolutionary time, we have unearthed invaluable insights about the beauty and potential of midlife.

Exploring the many facets of midlife within the book's pages, we've encountered a variety of situations and viewpoints that contribute to this stage's distinctiveness and fulfillment. From appreciating the experiences that have shaped us to welcoming change and healing, each component has provided a unique lens through which to view the priceless opportunities that midlife offers.

Gratitude emerges as a central theme, inviting us to consider our path thus far and offer gratitude for the blessings in our lives. Acknowledging the abundance of our experiences, relationships, and lessons gained gives us a deeper sense of contentment and joy that enables us to fully live in the now.

Feeling passionate about midlife also means urgently embracing change and replenishing. We get the chance to reflect on who we are, look for new hobbies, and welcome new experiences as we investigate the changes that come with growing older. Rather than fearing change, we should embrace it as an opportunity for growth and transformation that may unpredictably advance our path.

Additionally, midlife provides us with the chance to concentrate on our wealth and pursue activities that bring us joy and fulfillment. Midlife provides us with the time and space to concentrate on our happiness and success, whether it be by spending quality time with friends and family, engaging in leisure activities, or making investments in self-care.

In addition to self-awareness, midlife also presents opportunities for strengthening relationships with others. Midlife is a chance to build meaningful relationships that improve our lives and provide us with support and friendship along the way, whether it's strengthening current ties or creating new ones.

Thinking back on our journey together, it's clear that reaching midlife fever involves more than just living in the moment; it also involves looking forward with excitement and idealism to what lies ahead. We can truly experience our brilliant years without boundaries if we embrace the opportunities that come with reaching midlife and fully utilize their potential.

Rebecca, a woman in her late forties, talks about her incredible participation in **Amber N. Spruill** book "Becoming Hopelessly Enamored with

**Falling In Love With Midlife**

Midlife: Opening 15 Motivations to Cherish Life in Your Brilliant Years." Having initially been anxious about entering this stage of life, Rebecca was pleasantly surprised by the meaningful events and compelling points of view presented in the book.

Rebecca was greatly awakened and inspired to greet midlife with optimism and enthusiasm by the book's emphasis on appreciation and practical advice, as well as its captivating narrative. After putting the techniques the book outlined into practice, Rebecca saw significant improvements in her overall prosperity and fulfillment. This led her to recommend the book to anybody considering the challenges and opportunities of midlife.

As we approach the outer limits of our research on midlife, it is important to think about how we can honor this important stage of life. Honoring midlife is more than just marking the passage of time; it's also about acknowledging the experiences, role models, and growth that have shaped us. Praise for reaching midlife, whether in group settings with loved ones or private meditation, enables us to honor the path we've already taken and welcome the opportunities that lie ahead with contentment and hope.

More than just a book, "How to Love Midlife: Unlocking 15 Reasons to Loving Life in Your Golden Years," is a manual for embracing the grandeur, possibilities, and extravagance of midlife. I hope that the stories and insights found inside these pages inspire you to cherish this revolutionary stage of life and fall in love with midlife all over again.